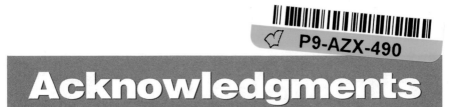

Acknowledgments

The authors gratefully acknowledge the invaluable assistance of our acquisition editor, Ted Miller, and our developmental editor, Elaine Mustain; and our secretaries, Susan Ramsden and Linda Tranisi. We are most appreciative of our photographer, Sharon Townson, and our exercise models, Diane Caledonia, Dick Carey, Robert Concannon, George Conway, Ian Dargin, Marie Hegerty, Herb Kirshnit, Fran Ramsden, Verna Trotman, Skip Tull, and Warren Westcott. Thanks also to Debra Wein, R.D., for her sound advice on eating for strength in Chapter 9, and to Steve Block, President of SPRI Products, Inc., for providing the elastic bands used in the exercise illustrations in chapter 10. Special thanks to the Executive Directors of the South Shore YMCA, Ralph Yohe, Mary Moore, and William Johnson. Most of all we appreciate the support of our wives, Claudia Westcott and Susan Baechle, and God's grace as we combined our efforts to produce this practical strength-training book.

Introduction

Better Years Ahead Through Strength Training

Muscles are the engines of the body. Unfortunately, muscles lose size and strength with age, resulting in physical weakness and a variety of degenerative problems. Good news! You can largely avoid muscle loss by doing regular strength training. Better news! You can replace muscle tissue you've already lost regardless of your age. Great news! You can replace a rather large amount of lost muscle in a relatively short time through a simple strength-training exercise program.

We recently completed a five-year study, examining the effects of regular strength training on previously sedentary adults and seniors. A total of 1,132 men and women participated in our two-month fitness program, which featured 30 minutes of strength training on 12 resistance machines two or three days a week. On average, the younger adults (21 to 40 years) and the middle-aged adults (41 to 60 years) added 2.3 pounds of muscle, and the older adults (61 to 80 years) added 2.4 pounds of muscle. That's right—the oldest participants responded similarly to strength-training exercises as those who were younger!

But what happens after the eight-week training program? Aren't people tired of all that weight lifting? Don't they go back to the couch-potato existence as soon as possible? Not at all. As a result of their physical improvements, 95 percent of the program participants continued to strength train and experienced further muscle development. For example, after 18 months of strength-training exercises, Dick Carey (age 60) added 5 pounds of muscle, lost 17 pounds of fat, and increased the speed of his golf swing.

Was Mr. Carey in better condition to start with than you are? Probably not, and our research shows that being out of shape does not diminish your strength-training benefits. For example, the men in this study were divided into five fitness categories, based on their initial percent body fat. Although all the program participants made impressive improvements, those starting in the less fit categories added the most muscle, lost the most fat, and experienced the greatest reduction in resting blood pressure. In other words, those who needed strength-training exercises the most, benefited the most!

But what about older adults, such as those in their 80s? George Conway had been physically inactive until he turned 80, when he began walking and doing strength-training exercises at the YMCA. Now 94, Mr. Conway is strong and fit and the holder of several age-group world records in racewalking. There is simply no age limit on strength training and muscle building. In fact, in a study at Tufts University, 90-year-old women increased muscle mass by 9 percent and physical strength by more than 100 percent as a result of regular strength training.

Speaking of women, two out of three participants in our research program were female, and most had never tried strength-training exercises before. But after only eight weeks of training, they replaced almost two pounds of muscle and increased overall strength by more than 40 percent. These changes also resulted in major improvement in functional capacity and physical performance capabilities of the women in this study.

So the previously sedentary adults did strength training, but they didn't like it, right? Wrong! After completing the program they rated their strength-training experience an average of 4.9 on a 5-point scale. We are sure that you, like our participants, will be pleased with both the process and the product of sensible strength-training exercises.

What if you have done strength-training exercises before and know all about bench presses, curls, and squats? That is helpful, but there is a lot more to comprehensive muscle conditioning, especially when you're past 50. For example, when you were younger, you probably strength trained hard and attained excellent results. But you most likely spent a lot of time in the weight room, probably performed a few high-risk exercises, and may have experienced some overtraining effects. Keep in mind that a 20-year-old body is much more forgiving than an over-50 body. Although aging does not reduce your ability to gain strength and build muscle, it does make your body more susceptible to exercise-related injuries. This book is designed to help you regain your strength fitness safely and effectively. Feel free to move through the training program at a faster rate, but follow the exercise recommendations. You should find the progressive workout protocols highly productive and very time-efficient.

In this book, we'll present research-based guidelines to help you begin and maintain a sound strength-training program. The exercise procedures are safe and effective, the training sessions are brief and progressive, and the workouts start at your present level of strength fitness. Even so, be sure to check with your personal physician before putting on your sweat suit, especially if you have a history of cardiovascular, orthopedic, or neuromuscular problems. We encourage you to read every chapter and follow all of the exercise guidelines carefully for a successful and satisfying strength-training experience. As with all the success experienced by our students, we look forward to your successes, and you should too!

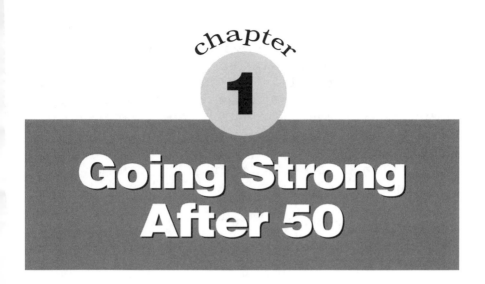

1

Going Strong After 50

You already know that strength training is the best way to build larger and stronger muscles. You have undoubtedly seen bodybuilders on magazine covers and heard football commentators report on the amount of weight key players can bench press. You may also be aware that lifting weights is an important component of athletic conditioning programs. In fact, you may have done some strength training as a sport team participant.

You may think, however, that only young or athletic individuals should use strength-training equipment. Indeed, many people tell us they feel that way. They pass by the strength-training facility and wish that they were in good enough shape to use the exercise equipment. But they need to understand that you don't get strong in order to do strength-training exercises—you do strength-training exercises to get strong.

Then again, you may be a seasoned strength trainer who has read muscle-building magazines and accumulated dozens of barbell plates. Although you know a lot about strength-training exercises, you should consider the needs of an older musculoskeletal system that is still responsive, yet more susceptible to overuse effects and training injuries. The exercise programs we'll present in this book provide both a safe and time-efficient approach to strength fitness. In fact, many committed strength-training exercisers have switched to our program because it produces excellent results, requires less training time, and carries a low risk of injury.

You may have heard that strength training is bad for your heart and raises your blood pressure, but that is most unlikely. In fact, research conducted at Johns Hopkins University reveals that sensible strength-training exercises are beneficial for cardiac rehabilitation patients and studies at the University of California show that properly performed strength training may actually reduce resting blood pressure.

Perhaps you are already overweight and fear that strength training will make you even heavier. Not so. Study after study has shown that strength-training exercises simultaneously increase muscle and decrease fat, resulting in a lower body weight and a healthier body composition.

Of course, it could be that you are simply too old to benefit from strength training . . . but don't count on it. Research with 60-, 70-, and 80-year-old men and women has demonstrated many physical improvements from a basic program of strength-training exercises. In fact, the *Journal of the American Medical Association* has reported significant gains in muscle strength and physical function in 90-year-olds who do strength-training exercises! As Dr. William Evans, one of the leading researchers on exercise and aging says, "You're never too old to exercise, but you're probably too old not to exercise."

Most likely, what you haven't heard about strength training is far more important and accurate than what you have heard. For starters, strength training can prevent the otherwise inevitable loss of muscle and reduction in metabolic rate that accompany the aging process. But what if you have already experienced significant muscle loss and metabolic slow-down? Good news! No matter what your age, you can replace muscle tissue and speed up your metabolism through regular strength training.

Myths to the contrary aside, strength training makes good sense from a medical perspective. That's right! Research indicates that strength training can reduce your risk of obesity, osteoporosis, diabetes, colon cancer, high blood pressure, unfavorable blood cholesterol, low back pain, and arthritic discomfort (Tufts University; University of Maryland; University of Florida).

No wonder almost all our adult exercise participants report feeling and functioning better after completing our eight-week strength-training program. So much better, in fact, that over 90 percent of them continue strength training as a regular part of their lifestyles.

Why You Should Strength Train

Here are 12 reasons every adult over 50 should make strength training a regular part of his or her lifestyle.

Maintain Your Muscle

When asked about strength training, many people respond that they have no desire to build big muscles. If only they knew how hard it is to develop large muscles and how few people have the genetic potential to do so! Rather than talking about too much muscle, we should be more concerned about too little muscle. Consider this fact of aging: Unless we exercise the muscles we have properly, we lose five to seven pounds of muscle tissue every decade of adult life. Because muscles are the engines of the body, this is similar to dropping from an eight-cylinder car, to a six-cylinder car, to a four-cylinder car, to a motor scooter.

This progressive muscle loss is responsible for two of life's major problems and is associated with a variety of health-related consequences. The first problem is that your capacity to function is reduced, which leads to less physical activity and further muscle loss. The second problem is reduced calorie use, which leads to a slower metabolism. A slower metabolism means that eating the same amount of food will result in the gradual accumulation of body fat.

Maintain Your Metabolism

Most people recognize that too much fat is a serious health threat, and many try to reduce their fat weight through low-calorie diets. Unfortunately, even though 40 percent of Americans are presently dieting, only 1 out of 20 will be successful.

Why? Because excess fat is only part of the problem, and losing fat is only part of the solution.

Although less obvious, the more important part of the problem is too little muscle. Due to muscle loss, your metabolism decreases by as much as five percent every decade of adult life. This is because every pound of muscle uses dozens of calories a day just to sustain itself. So when you lose muscle, the calories that were previously used to maintain metabolically active tissue now goes into fat storage. Fortunately, strength training helps maintain muscle tissue, thus increasing the metabolic rate, which means you'll have larger engines and less fat as you age.

Add Muscle Tissue

The really exciting news is that you are never too old to replace muscle tissue! Between the ages of 82 and 85 my [Wayne's] father added more than 12 pounds of muscle through strength training, and what a difference it has made in his activity level. In addition to caring for a large house and yard, he walks and cycles every day and enjoys a productive lifestyle as he approaches 88 years.

Our research with 1,132 previously sedentary adults shows that two months of strength training provides enough time to add a lot of muscle tissue. The men averaged 3.7 pounds more muscle and the women averaged 1.7 pounds more muscle. And they didn't spend all day in the weight room either! They achieved these results through 30-minute training sessions, only two or three days a week.

Increase Metabolic Rate

As you add muscle, you automatically increase your metabolism. Consider the additional muscle as engine cylinders that burn calories and produce energy. The more you have, the better off you are. Research on men and women over age 50 at Tufts University revealed that adding three pounds of muscle produced a seven percent increase in the resting metabolic rate. The reason: At rest a pound of muscle requires over 35 calories a day just for tissue maintenance. Compare this to only 2 calories a day used by a pound of fat. Therefore, the increase in muscle that results from strength training produces a higher level of calorie use every day. That's one reason why those of you who previously strength trained could eat a lot of food without adding fat when you were working out.

Reduce Body Fat

Let's assume you've already put on some fat that you want to lose. Many people will tell you to do endurance exercises such as walking or cycling to burn the extra calories. Endurance exercises can certainly help, but strength training is even more effective for reducing body fat.

Studies show that strength training increases both muscle mass and tissue activity, which in turn produces an accelerated metabolic rate and a higher daily energy expenditure. For example, the participants in Tufts' study increased their daily energy expenditure by 15 percent through just 30 minutes of strength-training exercises three days a week. Even though they ate about 350 more calories per day, the subjects lost an average of four pounds of fat over the 12-week training period.

Think about it! A basic strength-training program enabled men and women over age 50 to add muscle, reduce fat, and eat more food—all at the same time and in a safe and healthy manner.

Increase Bone Mineral Density

As you are probably aware, osteoporosis is a degenerative disease caused by a gradual loss of bone proteins and minerals. Because your muscle condition largely determines your bone condition, weak muscles lead to weak bones and strong muscles lead to strong bones. Numerous studies, including those at Tufts University and University of Maryland, have found that strength training helps to maintain bone strength, and therefore can serve as an excellent preventive measure against osteoporosis. Research has also demonstrated that strength training can increase bone mineral density in people of all ages, essentially reversing the bone-weakening processes. Although other factors, such as genetics, hormones, and nutrition, play important roles in your bone health, strength training is an activity that will develop a stronger musculoskeletal system and help your bones resist deterioration.

Improve Glucose Metabolism

Your ability to use glucose is closely related to your risk of adult onset diabetes. While exercise in general enhances glucose metabolism, strength training may benefit this process the most. Studies at the University of Maryland have demonstrated a 23 percent increase in glucose metabolism after only four months of strength training. This impressive improvement may be attributed to both the high energy demands of strength training and the greater metabolic requirements of larger and stronger muscles. Although more research is necessary, at this time it appears that regular strength training should help decrease the likelihood of developing adult onset diabetes.

Speed Up Food Transit

It takes time to move food through your gastrointestinal system, and research indicates that slow transit times increase the risk of colon cancer. Is it possible to speed up your digestive processes? Yes. A recent study at the University of Maryland revealed a 56 percent increase in gastrointestinal transit after only three months of strength training. Now that is good news on several fronts!

Lower Blood Pressure

Contrary to conventional wisdom, sensible strength training does not raise your resting blood pressure. Whether you do strength-training exercises alone or in combination with endurance exercises, it can result in lower resting blood pressure. For example, our study involving more than 250 men and women over age 50 showed a four percent reduction in resting blood pressure after eight weeks of standard strength and endurance exercises. Of course, you should train sensibly and breathe properly to maintain a desirable blood pressure response while doing strength-training exercises.

Improve Blood Lipids

Blood lipids include high-density lipoproteins (the good cholesterol), low-density lipoproteins (the bad cholesterol), and triglycerides (the storage form of fat). Although genetic makeup plays a major role in this area, both diet and exercise may positively influence your blood lipid levels. While some research has shown no effect, several studies have demonstrated better blood lipid levels after regular strength training. The combination of strength training, aerobic activity, and less fat in your diet may be the best way for you to create a more desirable blood lipid profile.

Maintain or Improve Low Back Health

Although it sounds too bad to be true, medical professionals estimate that four out of five American adults experience low back pain. Studies indicate a direct relationship between weak low back muscles and low back problems. Fortunately, as you strengthen your low back muscles, you reduce your risk of low back pain. In fact, research at the University of Florida Medical School reveals that 80 percent of their low back patients have significantly less discomfort after several weeks of systematic strength training. Why? Well-conditioned muscles provide better support and shock absorption, which prepares the low back muscles to absorb forces that might otherwise overstress the sensitive components of your spinal column.

Reduce Arthritic Pain

If you have arthritis, you may be avoiding strength-training exercises—and understandably so. But some research suggests stronger muscles may be helpful for improving joint function and easing arthritic discomfort. Although the exact mechanisms are not fully understood, studies at Tufts University have shown a reduction in arthritic pain following a program of regular strength training.

Strength Training Is for You

You are now aware of several convincing reasons to get involved in a strength-training program. You may feel, however, that the people who participate in strength-training studies are somehow different from yourself. You probably assume that they have a pretty high fitness level to start with, right? Not usually. In fact, most of the 1,132 adults who have participated in our strength research programs over the past five years were previously inactive, overweight, and out of shape. Yet, on average, after just two months of training, they added 2.4 pounds of muscle, lost 4.6 pounds of fat, and increased strength by 43 percent. They also lowered resting blood pressure by 4 percent and increased joint flexibility by 16 percent.

All of these outcomes help make everyday tasks requiring physical effort easier to do and participation in recreational activities more successful. For example, a large group of golfers averaging 52 years of age improved their driving power by four percent after completing our strength-training program. Many of these were former athletes who had become too busy to exercise, sliding into a sedentary lifestyle. But after seeing the results of the strength-training program, they assured us that this would never happen again.

We hope you are now convinced that regular strength training can help you look better, feel better, and function better. Yet, you may still have concerns about the safety of strength training. After all, isn't weight lifting a high-risk activity? Not if you apply the training principles and follow the exercise procedures we'll present in the following chapters. In fact, the injury rate among our adult strength-training exercisers is extremely low, and as long as you remember not to do too much too soon, you'll probably fare well, too. To reduce the chances of injury, we'll provide special guidelines for those starting with low strength. Simply look for the boxes that say "For Lower Strength Levels."

So, should every adult buy a set of barbells? That is one option, but you may prefer the efficiency of well-designed strength-training machines. We'll show you how to exercise properly with both free weights and resistance machines as well as some other training alternatives. And for you who have strength trained in the past, we will present productive programs for safely regaining your muscular fitness.

Are There Any Good Reasons Not to Strength Train?

Perhaps you have heard how much time some athletes put into their strength and conditioning programs, and you don't want any part of a two-hour weight workout. Don't worry! Strength training need not be a time-consuming activity. Remember, essentially all the benefits we've reported in this chapter were achieved by doing less than 30 minutes of strength training, two or three days per week. Because muscle development depends more on exercise intensity than workout duration, brief training sessions can produce excellent results. One hour a week is all the time you need to attain a high level of strength fitness.

But isn't strength training boring? Definitely not! You will do about a dozen different resistance exercises, each performed in a different movement pattern. You will spend only 50 to 70 seconds performing each strength-training exercise, hardly enough time to become bored. And the challenge of completing exercises in proper form should keep you focused. In fact, the sense of satisfaction that will accompany each strength-training session should make your workout an interesting part of your day.

Medical Clearance: An Important First Step

As you can see, the reasons for strength training are compelling, and the rationalizations to avoid this beneficial activity are very weak. But of course you should talk with your personal physician before beginning any exercise program. Although it is unlikely that your doctor will tell you not to do strength training, you may have a preexisting condition that will require some modifications to the training programs we'll present in this book. So check with your physician and then commit yourself to a sensible strength-training program that can add years to your life and life to your years.

"Weight training has been an integral part of my competitive preparation for many years. Long ago, while competing in a high-risk predominantly male sport, I realized the way to victory was mental toughness and strength—which in turn enabled me to endure the rigors of cross-country motorcycle racing on a national level. At the age of 50 I was able to win a national championship for downhill mountain biking and the bronze metal in cross-country—once again I turned to strength training to develop a base for my competitive season. As I am in a full-time battle with osteoarthritis, strength training has now become my key for athletic survival, although my doctors told me my arthritis was so severe that I ought to stop weight training altogether. I met the challenge by pre-exhausting muscles before specific lifting exercises. Now I am lifting as much as I did five years ago, and recent tests have shown that my bone density is excellent.

My goal is to achieve a third national championship and train for the long run! Weight training has been and will always be my foundation for excellence in sport and better health in life after 50."

—Marcia MacDonald, age 54

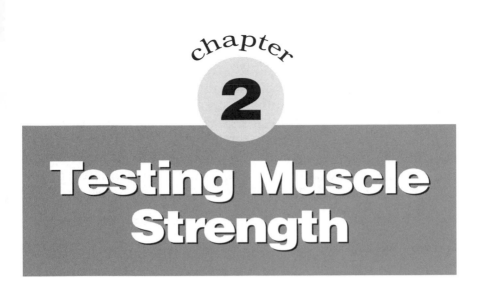

chapter

2

Testing Muscle Strength

Now that you're ready to begin your strength-training program, you need to establish an appropriate starting point. So in this chapter, we'll look at factors that influence your strength potential, procedures for assessing your current strength level, and guidelines for determining your starting weightloads.

Factors That Influence Your Strength Potential

The three most critical characteristics that affect your muscular fitness are your gender, age, and lifestyle.

Gender

It is no secret that men are stronger than women. For example, in our study of more than 900 middle-aged adults, the men were 50 percent stronger than the women in a standard test of leg strength. Does this mean that males have higher-quality muscle than females? Not at all. It simply means that men, who are typically larger, have more muscle mass than women. When compared on a muscle-for-muscle basis, however, the men and women in this study were equally strong. And other research reveals that men and women have similar rates of strength development. Although women typically use lighter weightloads, men and women gain strength and improve muscular fitness in a similar manner.

So the only real difference between men's and women's approaches to strength training is the amount of weight they should use, which can be seen in table 2.1. This table presents the average weightloads used by 134 men and women over age 50 for 13 standard Nautilus machine exercises after two months of strength training.

Age

As indicated by the exercise weightloads in table 2.1, strength decreases about 5 to 10 percent per decade in adults who do not exercise their muscles. This is due to the gradual loss of muscle tissue that accompanies the aging process. As we

Table 2.1

WEIGHTLOADS AFTER TWO MONTHS' STRENGTH TRAINING (IN POUNDS; 134 SUBJECTS)*

| | AGE GROUPS | | | | | |
| | 50-59 | | 60-69 | | 70-79 | |
	males	females	males	females	males	females
Leg extension	90.0	60.0	82.5	57.5	75.0	55.0
Leg curl	90.0	60.0	82.5	57.5	75.0	55.0
Leg press	180.0	120.0	160.0	110.0	140.0	100.0
Chest crossover	85.0	50.0	80.0	47.5	70.0	45.0
Chest press	87.5	50.0	80.0	47.5	72.5	45.0
Compound row	117.5	77.5	110.0	75.0	102.5	70.0
Shoulder press	82.5	42.5	72.5	40.0	62.5	37.5
Biceps curl	75.0	42.5	70.0	40.0	60.0	37.5
Triceps extension	75.0	42.5	70.0	40.0	60.0	37.5
Back extension	95.0	72.5	90.0	67.5	85.0	65.0
Abdominal curl	95.0	57.5	90.0	55.0	80.0	52.5

*Actual weightloads will be different on other resistance machines, but the strength relationships will be similar for men and women across the three age groups.

discussed in chapter 1, unless you strength train on a regular basis, you will probably lose more than five pounds of muscle every decade of adult life, and this will definitely lower your strength level.

Fortunately, regular training maintains and increases muscle strength. The 367 men and women represented in figure 2.1 increased muscle strength by an average of more than 40 percent during our eight-week exercise program, and the rate of strength gain was similar for all age groups.

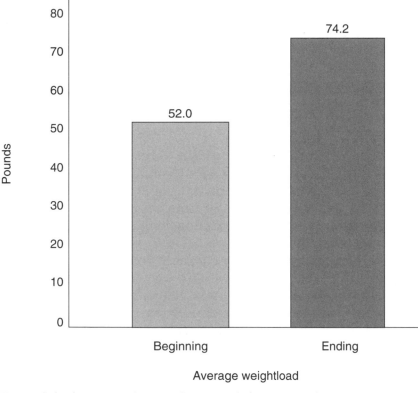

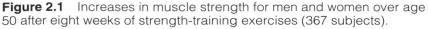

Average weightload

Figure 2.1   Increases in muscle strength for men and women over age 50 after eight weeks of strength-training exercises (367 subjects).

Lifestyle

Our research data provides reasonable estimates of average strength levels for men and women of various ages. It does not account for individual differences, however, such as general lifestyle and activity patterns. For example, if you have a physically demanding occupation, such as carpentry, you are likely to be stronger than your neighbor who is an accountant. Likewise, if you enjoy active hobbies, like gardening or hiking, you will probably be stronger than your friend who spends free time knitting.

While your general lifestyle and activity patterns don't limit your training benefits, they may influence your strength potential. You may never become as strong as your cousin who still works the farm, but you can become a lot stronger than you are now. And that is what really matters—personal physical improvement that enables you to look, feel, and function better.

Procedures for Assessing Your Strength Level

Remember when you were in high school and the physical education teacher evaluated your muscular fitness with push-ups and pull-ups? These body weight exercises were tough tests then, and they are totally unacceptable for most of us now. How many people do you know who can pull themselves up to the chinning bar?

Although strength training can help you perform push-ups and pull-ups, these body weight exercises are poor self-assessment tools. You'll get more relevant strength information from an evaluation that uses external resistance (weights), such as the YMCA leg extension test.

YMCA Leg Extension Test

The YMCA leg extension test is an appropriate strength assessment for adults of all ages. First, this strength evaluation is based on data from more than 900 men and women. Second, it addresses the large and regularly used thigh (quadriceps) muscles, making it a practical strength assessment. Third, this test uses a 10-repetition weightload, making it a safe strength assessment. As most people can complete 10 repetitions with 75 percent of their maximum resistance, the testing weightloads are well below their muscular limits and so pose a very low risk of injury. Fourth, the YMCA leg extension test evaluates muscular performance relative to body weight, making it a fair strength assessment for men and women of various body sizes. That is, you are evaluated on the percentage of your body weight that you can lift, rather than on the actual weightload. For example, a 100-pound woman who lifts 50 pounds achieves the same score as a 200-pound woman who lifts 100 pounds, as both lift 50 percent of their body weight.

The original strength classifications were derived from leg extension scores for men and women in their mid-40s. However, more recent research on strength changes during the midlife years provides modified performance standards for people in their 50s, 60s, and 70s. You should, therefore, find this test information very useful for determining your present strength level (see YMCA leg extension test score categories on page 16).

Test Procedures

- Begin by selecting a weightload on the leg extension machine that is about 25 percent of your body weight. (For exercise photo, see page 51). Complete 10 repetitions in the following manner:
  1. Lift the roller pad in two seconds until your legs are fully extended.
  2. Hold the fully extended position momentarily.
  3. Lower the roller pad in four seconds until the weightstack almost touches.
- Take a two-minute rest, select a weightload that is about 35 percent of your body weight, and again complete 10 repetitions in the prescribed manner.
- If successful, take a two-minute rest, select a weightload that is about 45 percent of your body weight, and again complete 10 repetitions in the prescribed manner.
- Continue testing in this manner with progressively more resistance until you find the heaviest weightload you can lift 10 times while maintaining proper form.
- Now divide this weightload by your body weight to obtain a strength score, which is used to assess your present level of strength fitness.

Evaluating Your Strength Fitness

After determining what percentage of your body weight you can use for 10 leg extensions, place your strength score in the appropriate category to assess your present level of strength fitness. For example: A 55-year-old male who weighs 180 pounds and completes 10 leg extensions with 120 pounds has a strength score of 66 percent, which ranks him in the above average category for quadriceps strength fitness. Or a 70-year-old female who weighs 120 pounds and completes 10 leg extensions with 60 pounds has a strength score of 50 percent—above average strength in her quadriceps.

YMCA LEG EXTENSION TEST SCORE CATEGORIES—MEN

Strength fitness	Ages 50-59	Ages 60-69	Ages 70-79
Low	44 or lower	39 or lower	34 or lower
Below average	45-54	40-49	35-44
Average	55-64	50-59	45-54
Above average	65-74	60-69	55-64
High	75 or higher	70 or higher	65 or higher

10 reps completed with 120 lbs.
120 lbs. divided by 180 lbs. = .66 = Above average for 55-year-old male

YMCA LEG EXTENSION TEST SCORE CATEGORIES—WOMEN

Strength fitness	Ages 50-59	Ages 60-69	Ages 70-79
Low	34 or lower	29 or lower	24 or lower
Below average	35-44	30-39	25-34
Average	45-54	40-49	35-44
Above average	55-64	50-59	45-54
High	65 or higher	60 or higher	55 or higher

10 reps completed with 60 lbs.
60 lbs. divided by 120 lbs. = .50 = Above average for 70-year-old female

Leg Squat Test

Although the YMCA leg extension test provides a good indication of your strength fitness, you may not have access to a Nautilus leg extension machine. If you do not, the leg squat test is an acceptable alternative. Like the YMCA leg extension test, this assessment targets your large and regularly used thigh (quadriceps and hamstrings) muscles. It is a practical method that you may perform anywhere without weight equipment. Because you use your own body weight for resistance, the results are personalized and require no mathematical calculations.

Test Procedures

- Begin by standing about 6 to 12 inches in front of a standard kitchen chair. Your feet should be about shoulder-width apart and your heels must remain on the floor (see figure 2.2 on page 18).
- Practice squatting down slowly until your buttocks lightly touch the chair seat. Cross your arms on your chest and keep your back as straight as possible.
- Do not let your knees extend forward farther than your toes.
- Once you are comfortable with the leg squat movement you may begin the strength test.
- Take four full seconds for the down phase of each leg squat and two full seconds for the up phase of each leg squat, making your buttocks lightly touch the chair seat during each repetition.
- Do as many perfect leg squats as you can without bouncing, experiencing pain, losing your balance, or going faster than six seconds per repetition.
- Place the number of leg squats you complete in the appropriate strength fitness category (see leg squat test score categories on pages 18-19).

Evaluating Muscle Strength

After performing as many leg squats as you can comfortably complete, compare that number with those in the appropriate

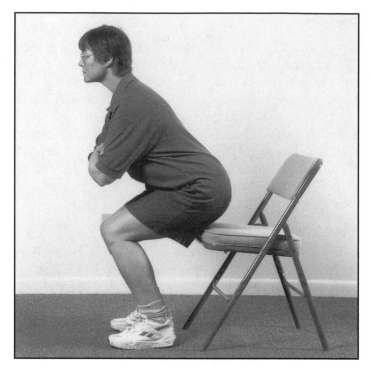

Figure 2.2   The leg squat test is a way to assess your strength without using a leg extension machine.

categories to estimate your present level of strength fitness. For example: A 62-year-old male who completes 16 leg squats has an average level of strength fitness in his thigh (quadriceps and hamstrings) muscles. Or a 58-year-old female who completes 19 leg squats has a high level of strength fitness in her thigh (quadriceps and hamstrings) muscles.

LEG SQUAT TEST SCORE CATEGORIES—MEN

Strength fitness	Ages 50-59	Ages 60-69	Ages 70-79
Low	12-14 reps	9-11 reps	6-8 reps
Below average	15-17 reps	12-14 reps	9-11 reps
Average	18-20 reps	15-17 reps	12-14 reps
Above average	21-23 reps	18-20 reps	15-17 reps
High	24-26 reps	21-23 reps	18-20 reps

LEG SQUAT TEST SCORE CATEGORIES— WOMEN

Strength fitness	Ages 50-59	Ages 60-69	Ages 70-79
Low	6-8 reps	3-5 reps	0-2 reps
Below average	9-11 reps	6-8 reps	3-5 reps
Average	12-14 reps	9-11 reps	6-8 reps
Above average	15-17 reps	12-14 reps	9-11 reps
High	18-20 reps	15-17 reps	12-14 reps

After completing the YMCA leg extension test or the leg squat test, you should have a reasonable estimate of your strength fitness. Although strength levels may vary among muscle groups, your leg assessment tests should, in general, provide a good indicator of your overall strength fitness. Keep in mind that the purpose of these assessments is not to discourage you, but to help you begin your training program with the appropriate exercise resistance.

Guidelines for Determining Your Starting Weightloads

In chapter 7, we'll present sample strength-training workouts that are based on your starting strength fitness assessment. The higher your strength level, the more resistance you will use to begin the training exercises. For example, if you scored above average in the strength fitness test, you will start training with heavier weightloads than if you scored below average.

As a general guideline, each strength fitness category represents a 2.5-pound greater training resistance than the next lower category. Let's say your strength fitness score was "average" and your recommended starting weightload in the chest press exercise is 50 pounds. If you scored "below average," you would begin with 47.5 pounds; and if you scored "low," you would begin with 45 pounds. But if you scored "above average," you would start with 52.5 pounds; and if you scored "high," you would start with 55 pounds.

For Lower Strength Levels

If your test results indicate that your strength fitness level is "very low," reduce the recommended starting resistance by 10 pounds or more.

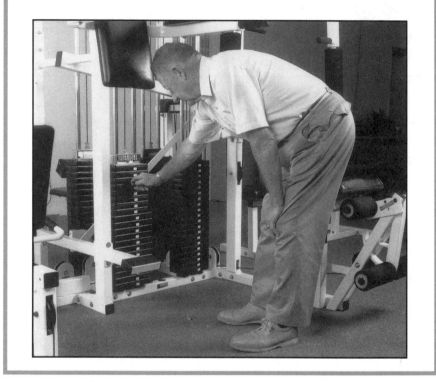

Of course, the recommended starting weightloads are also based on your age and gender. That is, older individuals will begin with less resistance than younger participants, and women will begin with lower weightloads than men.

If you take all these factors into consideration, the suggested starting weightloads should be appropriate. Still, due to individual differences, some of the recommended resistances may be too heavy and others may be too light. If you cannot correctly complete at least 8 repetitions of an exercise, you must reduce the resistance. If you can do more than 12 repetitions of an exercise, always maintaining correct form, you should increase the weightload.

So does the system work? Yes, for most people and for most strength-training exercises. Simply keep in mind that the recommended beginning weightloads should be challenging but not overwhelming. That is, the resistance should be sufficiently heavy so you feel the effort, but not so heavy as to cause muscle discomfort. If this is not the case, then you should make minor adjustments in the suggested starting weightload.

If you are elderly or very weak, we recommend starting all of the strength-training exercises at the lowest level and progressing very gradually. But if you have recently strength trained, you may find the suggested exercise weightloads below your ability. Feel free to use more resistance, but only if your exercise form is perfect. Never sacrifice proper training technique for heavier weightloads.

"As a woman with severe osteoporosis, I have found that strength training for the past two years has been beneficial in a number of ways: I am stronger and my balance has been enhanced considerably. Before beginning the program, I had fallen four times; however, in the past year and a half I have not fallen once. This benefit alone is invaluable because my bones are brittle."

—Marie Hegarty, age 61

Strengthening Safely at 50+

Strength-training exercises are not as simple as they may appear. To ensure safe and productive strength-training experiences, you need to both prepare properly and conduct each training session properly. Be sure to:

- Obtain physician approval.
- Train in a spacious exercise area.
- Wear functional activity attire.
- Maintain a desirable fluid balance.
- Use appropriate training loads.
- Follow a sensible training progression.
- Use correct technique.
- Work with a spotter on appropriate exercises.
- Emphasize movement control.
- Develop good training habits.

Prepare Properly

Proper preparation means that you are physically capable of performing strength-training exercises and that you are mentally committed to doing so. You need to establish a consistent workout schedule and follow a sensible program of progressive strength training. That's where this book will be most useful.

For Lower Strength Levels

If you have problems with balance or are beginning at lower strength levels, we advise you to start your strength training program with machine workouts. Resistance machines allow you to do most of your exercise from a sitting or prone position, usually with back support; they generally limit you to movements that are unlikely to result in injury and to movement patterns that are appropriate for the target muscles; they eliminate the possibility of dropping barbells, dumbbells, or weight plates on yourself; and they don't require you to stoop to lift any equipment. Once your strength levels are high enough, and if your balance improves, you may use free weights as long as you use the standard safety precautions.

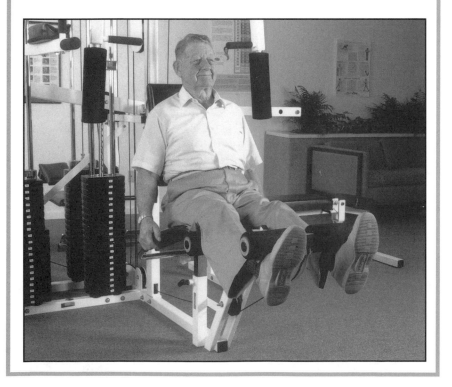

Physician Approval

As we mentioned in chapter 1, your physician should approve your strength-training activity. The questionnaire below will help you determine if you are physically ready to start strength training. Certain conditions may preclude your participation in a strength-training program. If you answer "yes" to any of the questions listed below, you must talk with your physician before beginning your strength-training workouts.

ASSESSING YOUR PHYSICAL READINESS

You should consult a physician before beginning a strength-training program if you answer "yes" to any of the following questions.

Yes	No	
___	___	Are you over age 50 (female) or 40 (male) and not accustomed to exercise?
___	___	Do you have a history of heart disease?
___	___	Has a doctor ever said your blood pressure was too high?
___	___	Are you taking any prescription medications, such as those for heart problems or high blood pressure?
___	___	Have you ever experienced chest pain, spells of severe dizziness, or fainting?
___	___	Do you have a history of respiratory problems, such as asthma?
___	___	Have you had surgery or experienced bone, muscle, tendon, or ligament problems (especially back or knee) that might be aggravated by an exercise program?
___	___	Is there a good physical or health reason not already mentioned why you should not follow a weight-training program?

T.R. Baechle, and R.W. Earle, 1995, *Fitness Weight Training*. (Champaign, IL: Human Kinetics), 24.

Spacious Exercise Area

Accidents are rare among adult strength trainers, but crowded exercise areas can increase the likelihood that they will occur. If you wish to train at a fitness center, choose one that has plenty of space between the strength-training machines and free-weight equipment. Avoid facilities that have cluttered floors, as items underfoot increase the potential for injury. In addition, too many people in the exercise room can hinder your concentration, possibly leading to mishaps.

If you train at home, find a spacious area to set up your exercise equipment and specific places to store your weights. Make sure you have ample lighting and air ventilation. Setting up workout equipment in a corner of a cluttered room can make your training sessions less enjoyable and create safety problems, especially if the exercise area is too small.

Spacious Exercise Area = No Clutter

Functional Activity Attire

Strength training is a challenging physical activity and as such requires functional exercise clothes. This begins with support-

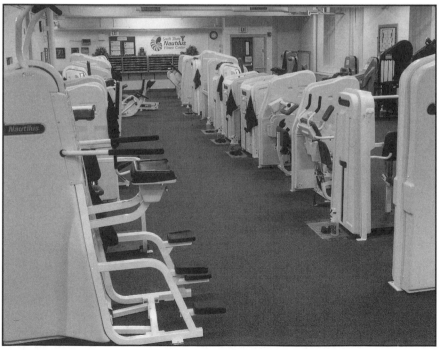

Figure 3.1a   Choose a fitness center that has plenty of space between the equipment.

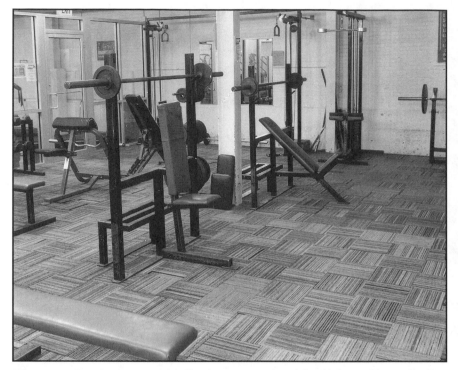

Figure 3.1b   A cluttered facility increases the risk of injury. Choose an uncluttered facility like the one shown here.

ive athletic shoes that provide good traction to prevent slipping. It also includes a loose-fitting pair of shorts and a T-shirt or a lightweight warm-up suit. Loose and light exercise clothes enable you to easily transfer body heat to the environment, avoiding undesirable rises in body temperature. Proper activity wear also gives you freedom of movement, allowing you to move comfortably without restriction through a full range of exercise actions.

Activity Attire = Safer and more comfortable training

Desirable Fluid Balance

Because our thirst mechanism becomes less sensitive as we age, most adults drink too little fluid for optimum health and physical function. Of course, exercise raises your fluid requirements due to increased energy metabolism and perspiration.

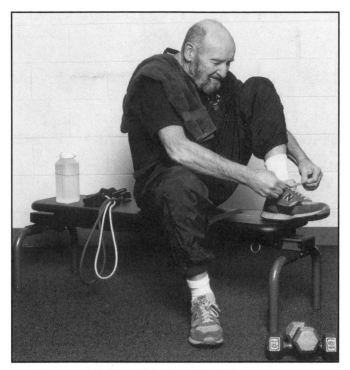

Figure 3.2   Proper clothing allows freedom of movement through a full range of exercise actions.

And people who strength train require even more fluid for muscle building, because muscle tissue is 80 percent water. If you are not sure that you are consuming enough water, simply check the color of your urine. If it is clear, you are well-hydrated, but if it is yellow, you may not be taking in sufficient fluids.

The best fluid is water, which you should drink throughout the day. At work, take a few swallows of water every time you pass the drinking fountain. At home, fill a bottle with water and sip it periodically while you are in the house or yard. Keep in mind that it is hard to drink too much water, but it is easy to take in too little.

Of course, you can substitute other beverages such as fruit juices, which provide important electrolytes, or low-fat milk, which is an excellent source of calcium. Carbonated beverages are acceptable, but we don't recommend fluids containing caffeine or alcohol because they act as diuretics.

You should have at least eight glasses of fluids daily. In addition, be sure to drink before, during, and after your strength-training sessions.

Fluid Balance = Eight or More Glasses of Fluids Each Day

Conduct the Workout Properly

This is where "the rubber meets the road." What you do during your workout determines how safe and productive your strength-training experience will be. So let's examine the factors that can both reduce your injury risk and increase the strength benefits.

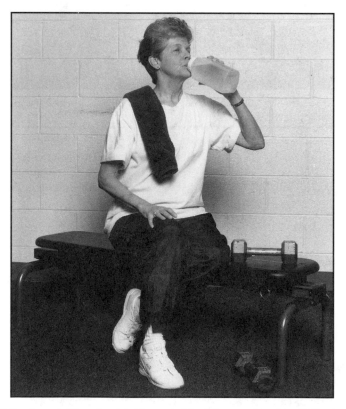

Figure 3.3 In addition to drinking eight glasses of water daily, be sure to drink before, during, and after your strength-training sessions.

Appropriate Training Loads

The first safety concern for all strength trainers is to select an appropriate exercise resistance. As we asserted in chapter 2, your beginning weightloads must not be too heavy. Even though most of the suggested starting weightloads should be appropriate, a few may require more muscle effort than you want to give. If so, simply reduce the weightload to where you can complete 8 to 12 repetitions in good form and without discomfort.

Appropriate Training Load = 8 to 12 Repetitions With
Good Form

Sensible Training Progression

As you become accustomed to strength training, you will be able to exert greater muscular effort and lift heavier loads. Just be sure to progress gradually so that you avoid doing too much too soon. This may be best accomplished by following the *2.5-pound rule*. That is, never increase your exercise training load by more than 2.5 pounds at a time. For example, if you are doing biceps curls with 25 pounds, increase the resistance to 27.5 pounds, rather than to 30 or more pounds.

But how do you know when to increase the resistance? Try using the *12-rep rule*. When you can correctly complete 12 repetitions of an exercise, you are ready to increase the training load (by 2.5 pounds). To be on the safe side, we recommend that you complete 12 repetitions of an exercise on two consecutive workouts before raising the weightload by 2.5 pounds. By practicing both the 2.5-pound rule and the 12-rep rule, you should minimize your risk of injury and maximize your training progression. This system has an outstanding safety record and typically produces over 40 percent strength increases after only two months of training.

Sensible Progression = 2.5-Pound Increase After 12
Repetitions During Two Consecutive Workouts

Correct Technique

Knowing how much weight to lift is essential, but knowing how to lift the weight is even more important. Exercise form and training safety are two sides of the same coin. To best avoid injuries and build stronger muscles, you must use proper training technique. In chapter 5, we'll explain and illustrate proper training technique for both resistance machine and free-weight exercises. As you can see in figure 3.4, *a* and *b*, improper lifting technique can place excessive stress on the low back. Please read the training instructions carefully and practice perfect form on every exercise repetition.

Correct Technique = Injury Prevention

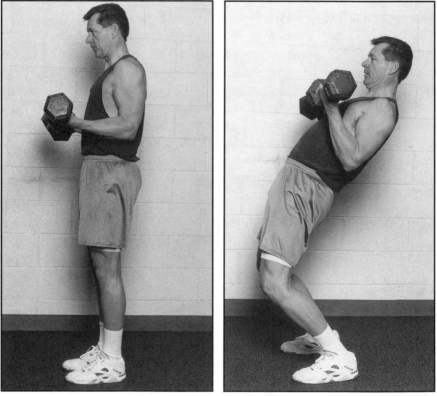

a.   *b.*

Figure 3.4   There is a right way (*a*) and a wrong way (*b*) to exercise. Improper lifting technique can place excessive stress on the low back.

Work With a Spotter

Some free-weight exercises such as the barbell bench press, barbell squat, and barbell heel raise increase your risk of injury due to the positioning of the barbell and the movement pattern. For example, if you are unable to complete the last repetition in the barbell bench press exercise and cannot place the barbell back on the standards, it rests on your chest which can be uncomfortable and may even injure you.Therefore, you must have a spotter present to assist you in these barbell exercises should you require help.

The spotter may help you lift the bar from the standards to start the exercise and can offer encouragement and technique comments as you perform the exercise. However, the most important function of the spotter is to assist you if you have difficulty controlling the barbell or completing the lift, thus protecting you from getting injured. For safety's sake be sure to have a competent and attentive spotter assist whenever you do barbell bench presses, squats, heel raises, or other exercises that may be difficult to perform or dangerous to do alone. In this book, we have placed an icon (⊖) beside the name of every exercise in which a spotter is necessary. It is very important that you take this information seriously and use a spotter where we have suggested that you do so.

Spotter = Safer Training

Movement Control

Good form applies to your upward and downward movements as you carefully lift and lower the weightloads. Both exercise components contribute to strength development, but lowering movements have a higher injury risk due to gravity, which tends to accelerate downward actions. So be sure to lift the resistance slowly and to lower the resistance even more slowly. A good rule of thumb is two seconds for each lifting movement and four seconds for each lowering movement. This way you always control the weightload, and gravity can't get the best of you on the way down.

Movement Control = Slow Lifting and Slower Lowering

Develop Good Training Habits

Developing good training habits helps you avoid injury and obtain the most from your exercise program. Don't forget that resistance exercise places stress on your muscles, so that jumping right into your weight workout is not a good idea. Always take a few minutes before each workout to warm-up, preparing your muscles for vigorous activity.

Even more importantly, be sure to end your exercise session with a gradual cool-down. This gives you a smooth transition from activity to rest, helping your heart ease back to normal circulation.

Walking and cycling are excellent warm-up and cool-down activities. Do four to six minutes of either activity at a low effort level, following this with some gentle stretching exercises.

Be cautious with your training procedures. Develop the habit of double-checking the little things. For example, if you use machines, make sure that you set your seat properly and select the correct weightload. Always fasten the seat belt if one is provided to ensure proper body alignment. If you use free weights, secure the locks carefully and use your legs rather than your back when taking or returning dumbbells and barbells from and to the floor. Be sure to use proper exercise technique and never struggle to complete an additional repetition.

Finally, always respect your body. Don't get into the habit of training if you are feeling below par or have muscle soreness. If you experience muscle or joint discomfort for more than a couple days, check with your physician before your next workout. One of the most important things you can do is to maintain a regular exercise program so that your muscles progressively become stronger. Missed sessions, other than for illness, invariably lead to training setbacks.

While strengthening your muscles is the key to better fitness and health, you should always train on the safe side. By following the recommendations in this book and developing good training habits, you should enjoy your strength-training exercises and experience a very low risk of injury in the process.

Developing Good Training Habits = Training by the Book

You are now aware of key strength-training considerations from a health and safety perspective. However, before you begin your workouts, be sure to carefully read chapter 5 to learn the proper form for each strength-training exercise.

"About 8 months ago I was feeling very low. I would travel to Florida to see my grandchildren only to be crippled with arthritis and not be able to enjoy them. The morning after attending any performance, my hands would be so swollen from clapping I couldn't use them. I'd dance a couple of line dances, then be gasping for breath due to my asthma. The next day I would hardly be able to walk, never mind going up stairs. One day the company I work for had a 'Wellness Fair.' I stopped at the South Shore YMCA booth and signed up for the 'Keeping Fit' program. I have been doing that program three times per week ever since. I have recently started swimming four times a week and have not had an arthritis attack since I have been doing the Nautilus program and cardiovascular workouts, and my breathing has improved dramatically."

—Florence Ragussa, age 56

Selecting the Right Equipment

The strength-training equipment you see in this book represents only a few of the hundreds of equipment options that are available. And because there are so many equipment options, deciding which will meet your needs and also are affordable can be frustrating. We have based the recommendations presented in this chapter on the assumption that those who are new to strength training may not initially want to invest a lot of money in equipment. Finally, in this chapter we'll include checklists to help you use the equipment safely. But if you prefer not to purchase strength-training equipment at all, we'll describe other training alternatives in chapter 10.

Free-Weight Home Equipment Considerations

The least expensive and the most versatile type of equipment to purchase is free-weight equipment, including barbells and dumbbells. Free-weight equipment does not take up much space, and you can use it to perform hundreds of different exercises. The unrestrained movement patterns permitted by free-weight equipment allow your joints to move through their full ranges, both increasing your flexibility and improving your overall muscle coordination. These advantages help explain why 40 million Americans use free weights.

Dumbbells, Barbells, and Benches

Let's look, now, at the basic free-weight equipment you'll need if you choose this route. These include a set of dumbbells, a barbell, and a bench with supports.

The adjustable dumbbells shown in figure 4.1 enable you to assemble the loads you need by adding weight plates to the dumbbell bar and securing them with locks, which are fasteners that fit on the end of the bar. Make sure that the locks are easy to tighten and loosen and that you can rely on them to keep the weight plates securely on the bar.

What exactly should you look for? Before purchasing locks, determine how much strength it takes to tighten and loosen them. Then, check to see if the weight plates stay on the dumbbell bar when it is tilted at a 45-degree angle. Ask the salesperson to tilt a lightly loaded bar to see if the weight plates stay on the end of the bar. If you do not have the grip strength needed to easily use a particular lock or if the weight plates slide off when the bar is tilted, seek out a different type.

If you are willing to spend a little more money, the premolded or fixed-weight, solid dumbbells are easier to use than the adjustable dumbbells (see figure 4.1). Since you do not have to assemble or disassemble them between exercises, premolded dumbbells enhance training efficiency. The downside of this type of dumbbell is that you need to purchase a good number of them if you want to use different weightloads in your workouts—which you probably will. A more economical approach and one that will equip you with what is needed to complete all exercises in the 10-week program described in chapter 7, is to purchase two adjustable dumbbells and the weight plates listed in "Basic Dumbbell Set Equipment". Two dumbbells and the 75 pounds in weight plates provide 15 different load options, ranging from 2.5 to 39.5 pounds (on each dumbbell assuming an unloaded bar weighs 2 lbs.) for approximately $40. The equipment listed will easily accommodate your dumbbell equipment needs.

BASIC DUMBBELL SET EQUIPMENT

A basic adjustable dumbbell set includes the following:

2 dumbbell bars with locks and

4 of each of the following:

10-pound plates

5-pound plates

2.5-pound plates

1.25-pound plates

Barbells

The barbell you select should be five or six feet in length unless you prefer an Olympic barbell set (figure 4.1). As with dumbbells, easy-to-use but secure locks are essential (figure 4.1). So apply the same convenience and safety criteria when selecting barbell locks. Listed below are the weight plates that comprise a basic 110-pound barbell set, plus two 1.25-pound plates that will create more load options. The bar and plates listed create 16 load options at a cost of approximately $70.

BASIC BARBELL SET

A basic barbell set includes the following:

1 5- to 6-foot barbell with locks and

4 of each of the following:

10-pound plates

5-pound plates

2.5-pound plates

1.25-pound plates

Weight Plates

The weight plates typically available for use in the home range from 1.25 to 25 pounds (figure 4.1).

Weight Benches

Weight benches are typically of two different types. One is designed without uprights (flat bench, figure 4.2), and the other with uprights (bench press bench, figure 4.2). Each

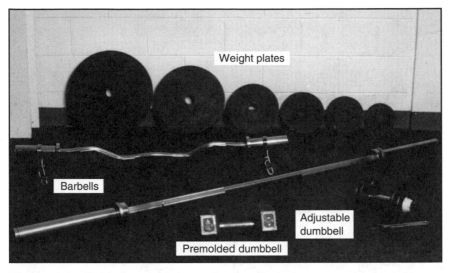

Figure 4.1 Basic free-weight equipment includes a set of adjustable dumbbells and/or fixed-weight dumbbells, locks, weight plates, and barbells.

bench enables you to perform a variety of chest, arm, and shoulder exercises while lying on your back or while sitting. If you intend to take on one of the advanced free-weight programs (chapter 8), you'll need a bench press bench to do the chest pressing exercises with a barbell. The uprights on the bench press bench have supports that provide you with a safe place for the barbell to rest. Please note that a flat bench will work fine for the basic free-weight workouts presented in chapter 7.

For a little more money you can purchase a bench that will adjust to different angles (incline bench) as shown in figure 4.2. Because you can change it to various seat positions, it is the most versatile type of bench.

What else might you need? The squat rack shown in figure 4.2 is a piece of free-weight equipment that enables you to include excellent exercises for the legs (squats) and shoulders (overhead presses) safely without spotters. Unless you have two qualified spotters, you will need to purchase a squat rack if you decide to include the squat exercise in the advanced training programs in chapter 8.

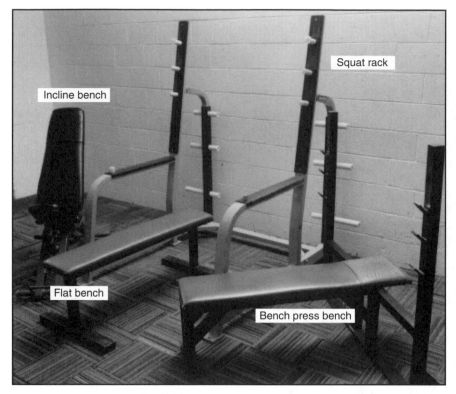

Figure 4.2 A variety of exercises may be performed on weight benches (shown are an incline bench, flat bench, bench press bench, and squat rack, which provides a safe resting place for the barbell and weights).

Free-Weight Equipment Costs

We present the equipment requirements and costs associated with performing the free-weight exercises in chapters 7 and 8 on page 39. The chart also includes costs associated with some optional equipment that may be of interest to you. As indicated in this chart, the cost of the dumbbells and bench for the 10-week program (chapter 7) is approximately $140, and the additional cost for equipment needed to do the workouts in chapter 8 is $550. The purchase of such equipment can give you several training options in your home for a relatively small initial investment. In comparison, a quality, easy-to-use, and versatile strength-training machine costs $1,000 to $2,000.

BASIC AND OPTIONAL EQUIPMENT COSTS

Basic equipment:

For the 10-week program in chapter 7, you'll need

2 adjustable dumbbells with locks and 75 pounds in weight plates	$ 40
1 flat bench	$ 100
	$ 140

For the advanced programs in chapter 8, you'll also need

1 5-foot barbell with locks and 87.5 pounds in weight plates	$ 70
1 bench press bench (with uprights)	$ 100
c. 1 squat rack	$ 380
	$ 550

Optional equipment:

1 set of premolded (solid) dumbbells (2- , 5-, 10-, 15-, 20-, 25-pound pairs)	$ 70
1 adjustable bench (substitute for other benches)	$ 130

Free-Weight Equipment Safety

If you decide to purchase and exercise with free-weight equipment, use the following checklist to safely get the most training benefit out of your equipment.

FREE-WEIGHT CHECKLIST

Before and During Training Sessions

___ Always load ends of bars in an even manner.

___ Always tighten loose locks securely.

___ Store weight plates appropriately so you don't trip over them.

___ Ensure that the bench is stable.

Machine Home Equipment Considerations

The popularity of weight training among men and women, which now exceeds 60 million participants in the United States, has spawned tremendous development of weight-training machines, especially for home gym use. Machine exercises are designed for ease of performance. You can change weightloads quickly and movement patterns are consistent. Machines also provide support for the body, and some models automatically match the resistance to your strength.

Machine Characteristics

Well-designed machines place a consistent stress on the muscles by means of a cam, or other device, that creates a longer (figure 4.3*a*) or shorter (figure 4.3*b*) distance between the pivot point and where the force is being applied, called the "pivot point distance." The design of the cam or other device is an attempt to match the shortest pivot point distance with the most difficult range of the exercise and the longest pivot point

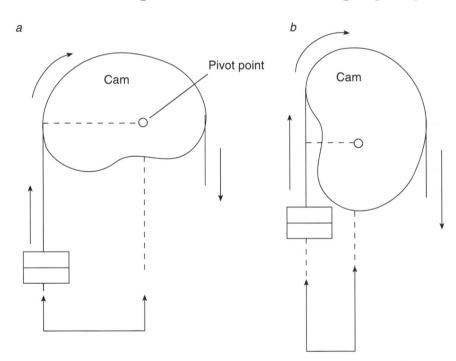

Figure 4.3 As the cam rotates from position *a* to *b*, the distance from the pivot point to the weight plate shortens, which has the effect of reducing the load, thereby resulting in a more uniform muscle effort throughout each repetition.

T.R. Baechle and B. Groves, 1992. Weight Training: Steps to Success. (Champaign, IL, Human Kinetics).

distance with the easiest range. Thus, the cam's shape attempts to match the "strength curve" (variation in strength throughout a range of movement) of the muscles involved in an exercise. In doing so, these machines approximate a muscle's force capability at each angle of movement, enabling it to maintain a more consistent level of effort throughout each repetition.

Free-weight exercises involve leverage changes that produce more resistance in some exercise positions and less in other positions. For example, as the dumbbell in figure 4.4 reaches level 3, the distance between the elbow and the dumbbell and the force required to continue curling are at their greatest points. When fatigue terminates a repetition in this exercise, failure usually occurs at level 3 even though you have sufficient strength to continue curling the dumbbell from points 1 to 2 and 4 to 5. Well-designed machines attempt to accommodate your muscles' force capability, enabling them to "contract through" the sticking point. When shopping for a machine, keep in mind that machines that use elastic resistance, such as those commonly advertised on television, may not adapt to your muscles' varying capabilities as well. Their advantages over machines with cams like those shown in figure 4.3, however, is that they are easy to move and store and are less expensive.

If you prefer to train on machines in your home consider the following points:

- How easy the exercises will be to learn
- Versatility—how many exercises you can perform on it
- Simplicity—how simple it is to set up for different exercises
- Equipment durability—quality of construction
- Convenience—ease of equipment assembly and disassembly
- Reputation of the equipment manufacturer
- Reputation of the local store from which you intend to purchase the equipment
- Costs of the equipment, including shipping and installation

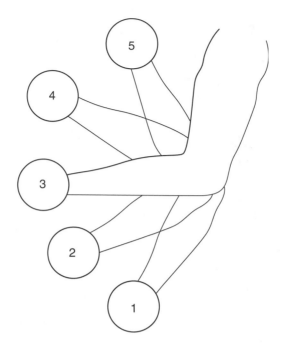

Figure 4.4   At position 3, the distance between your elbow and the dumbbell and the force required to complete the curl are at their greatest.

Machine Equipment Safety

If you decide to do machine training, use the following checklist to safely get the most out of your equipment. If any mechanical deficiencies exist, be sure to have them fixed before you use the equipment.

MACHINE CHECKLIST

Before and During Training Sessions

___ Check for frayed cables, belts, pulleys, worn chains, and loose pads.

___ Check for smooth movement of plates on guide rods.

___ Adjust levers and seats as needed.

___ Insert selector keys all the way into the weightstack.

___ Keep your hands away from the chains, belts, pulleys, and cams.

___ Never place your fingers or hands between weightstacks.

Training at a Fitness Facility

You may decide that you need the environment of a fitness facility to enjoy the workouts presented in this book. If so, the key factors to consider in choosing a training center are the

- qualifications of the fitness staff,
- services offered, and
- membership costs.

Ideally the facility you choose will be well-equipped and will have qualified professionals to develop and take you through an individualized training program. Typically, the facility will charge an initiation fee for a single membership of $70 to $250 ($85 to $300 for a family membership) and an annual fee of $275 to $580 ($345 to $670 for a family membership). In most facilities, personal training, day care, and other services are extra.

Selecting a Personal Trainer

A knowledgeable personal trainer can help you both enjoy and get the most out of the training programs presented in this book. A good personal trainer is capable of individualizing the workouts presented in this book and motivating you to make each workout count. He or she can also assist you when purchasing equipment for home use. An experienced personal trainer can give you advice about the equipment you need, help you identify a reputable retail store, and help you recognize a good deal. Your best approach to identify a

"Having passed my 70th birthday [and having suffered two herniated discs and a heart attack], I find that strength training allows me to maintain a full, active lifestyle. I now have the ability to engage in *all* activities I did in the past with ease and pleasure. I am more fit now than I have been in many years."

—**Herb Kirshnit, age 71**

personal trainer with these skills is to ask prospective trainers the following questions, then have them provide you with references from their current and previous clients.

- *What is your academic preparation related to personal training?*

  Look for course work associated with exercise physiology, biomechanics, nutrition, and ideally, a degree in exercise science, exercise physiology, physical therapy, athletic training, or physical education.

- *What certification credentials directly associated with personal training have you earned?*

  Look for nationally recognized credentials such as those offered by the National Strength and Conditioning Association or well-respected ones offered by organizations such as the American College of Sports Medicine or the American Council on Exercise.

- *How long have you been a personal trainer?*

  Look for someone who has been active in the business of personal training for at least two years. Be cautious about hiring an inexperienced personal trainer.

Before signing a contract with a personal trainer, it is a good idea to observe a prospective trainer working with a client. If you like what you see, it is still advisable to delay signing a contract until you train with him or her for at least one session. Also, consider the costs which typically range from $25 to $75 a session, and ask if the per session cost is less if you commit to a specified number of sessions.

Summary

Using equipment can add variety and enjoyment to your training, but is not a prerequisite to starting a strength-training program. If for whatever reason free-weight or machine equipment is not for you, consider the training alternatives we explain and illustrate in chapter 10. But if you decide to use machines or free-weight equipment, you should carefully consider the unique characteristics of each, and you should consult qualified professionals before purchasing equipment. Regardless of whether you include free-weight, machine, or alternative exercises, heed the safety checklists provided in this chapter. Finally, we encourage you to secure a qualified professional to assist you in the early phases of your strength-training program, but be sure to evaluate his or her credentials, services offered, costs, and comments from previous clients before signing a contract. We wish you success in making sound training decisions.

chapter

5

Using Correct Technique

We hope that by now you are convinced that strength training is for you and that you have decided which type of equipment you'll use. So what should you do with your new barbells or fitness facility pass? In this chapter, we'll explain how to correctly—and therefore safely—perform 39 exercises, carefully selected for past-50 strength trainers. Before beginning, however, be sure to read the next two chapters to learn the guidelines for safe and effective exercise (chapter 6) and the progressive pattern for a sound strength-training program (chapter 7).

For your convenience, we have organized the exercises into three major sections:

- lower body
- midsection
- upper body

Then we have further categorized the exercises by the specific muscle area they train (e.g., lower body: legs and calves). We have also listed the specific names of the primary muscles strengthened by each exercise. We hope that our organization of the exercises will make it easy for you to distinguish between machine and free-weight exercises and to

> This icon denotes exercises that require a spotter for safety (for more information on using spotters see chapter 3). Throughout this chapter certain exercises will be marked with this reminder. **Do not ignore this icon.** Types of exercises that require help from a spotter are those in which balance is a key factor and those in which a barbell may trap you, such as barbell bench presses and barbell squats. The barbell squat may be performed without a spotter if you use a squat rack with safety supports.

identify the names of exercises with the muscles they are intended to strengthen.

Use the anatomical drawings on the next two pages to learn the names of your muscles and their locations. Understanding where the muscles are as you exercise is important for two reasons:

- Research has shown that if you mentally focus on a specific muscle as you work it, your training will be more effective.

- Understanding muscle locations can help in your exercise selection to create balance among the muscle groups. If you over-exercise a muscle on one side of your body (for example, the quadricep) while under-exercising its opposing muscle (the hamstring) you will be more prone to injury in that muscle group. Triceps and biceps are another example of opposing muscles. Studying the drawings will help you identify other such pairings and groups.

Being aware of the specific muscle group combinations will help give you a visual reminder as well as a name for the area being strengthened. And this will help you get the most out of your workout.

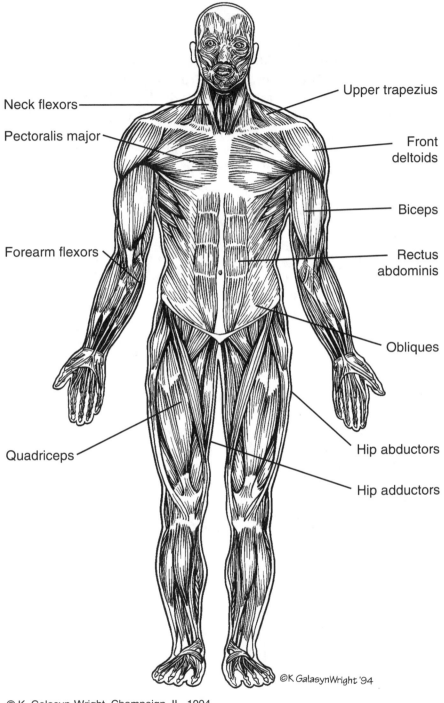

Neck flexors

Pectoralis major

Forearm flexors

Quadriceps

Upper trapezius

Front deltoids

Biceps

Rectus abdominis

Obliques

Hip abductors

Hip adductors

©K GalasynWright '94

© K. Galasyn-Wright, Champaign, IL, 1994

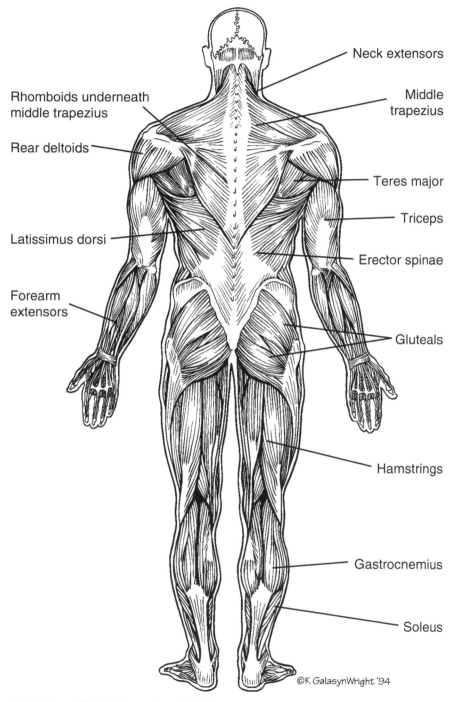

Neck extensors

Rhomboids underneath middle trapezius

Middle trapezius

Rear deltoids

Teres major

Triceps

Latissimus dorsi

Erector spinae

Forearm extensors

Gluteals

Hamstrings

Gastrocnemius

Soleus

©K. GalasynWright '94

© K. Galasyn-Wright, Champaign, IL, 1994

Lower Body Exercises

Below you will find 10 exercises which address the lower body. These include exercises for strengthening the legs, hips, and calves.

LEGS

Machine Leg Extension

quadriceps

Beginning Position

1. Adjust seat so knees are in line with machine's axis of rotation (where machine pivots). The axis of rotation is indicated by a red dot on Nautilus machines, which are shown in the following exercise illustrations.
2. Sit with back firmly against seat pad.
3. Position ankles behind roller pad, knees flexed about 90 degrees.
4. Grip handles.

Upward Movement Phase

1. Push roller pad slowly upward until knees are extended.
2. Exhale throughout upward movement.

Downward Movement Phase

1. Slowly return roller pad to starting position.
2. Inhale throughout lowering movement.

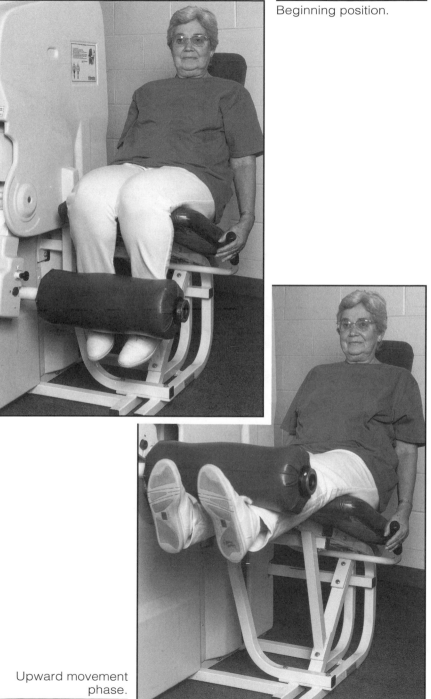

Beginning position.

Upward movement
phase.

Machine Leg Curl

hamstrings

Beginning Position

1. Adjust seat so knee joint is in line with machine's axis of rotation.
2. Sit with back firmly against seat pad.
3. Position lower legs between roller pads, knees extended.
4. Grip handles.

Backward Movement Phase

1. Pull roller pads slowly backward until knees are fully flexed.
2. Exhale throughout pulling movement.

Forward Movement Phase

1. Allow roller pads to return slowly to starting position.
2. Inhale throughout return movement.

LOWER BODY EXERCISES

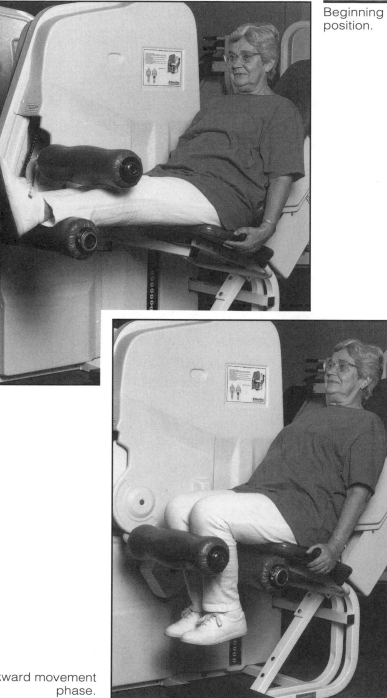

Beginning position.

Backward movement phase.

Free-Weight Dumbbell Squat

quadriceps, hamstrings, gluteals

Beginning Position

1. Grasp dumbbells using an underhand grip and stand erect with feet about hip-width apart and parallel to each other.
2. Position dumbbells with palms facing the outside surfaces of thighs.

Downward Movement Phase

1. Keep head up, eyes fixed straight ahead, shoulders back, back straight, and weight on entire foot throughout the upward and downward movement phases of this exercise.
2. Slowly squat down until thighs are parallel to floor.
3. Inhale throughout downward movement.
4. If balance is a problem, try positioning your upper back and buttocks against a wall for support (i.e., slide up and down a wall).

Upward Movement Phase

1. Begin upward movement by slowly straightening the knees and hips.
2. Exhale throughout upward movement.

LOWER BODY EXERCISES

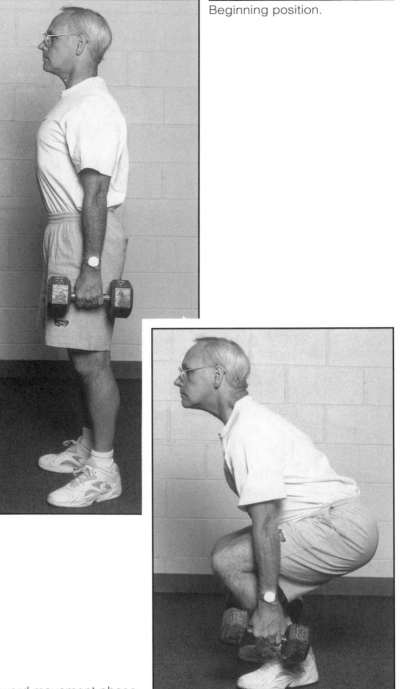

Beginning position.

Downward movement phase.

Free-Weight Barbell Squat

quadriceps, hamstrings, gluteals

Beginning Position

1. Position feet shoulder-width apart or wider and grip the bar overhand while it's on a rack.
2. Position bar on shoulders at base of neck, head up, eyes looking ahead.
3. Stand erect lifting bar out of rack.

Downward Movement Phase

1. Keep head up, eyes fixed straight ahead, shoulders back, back straight, and weight on entire foot throughout the upward and downward movement phases of this exercise.
2. Slowly squat down until thighs are parallel to floor.
3. Inhale throughout downward movement.

Upward Movement Phase

1. Begin upward movement by slowly straightening knees and hips.
2. Exhale throughout upward movement.
3. Carefully return the bar to rack after completing the set.

LOWER BODY EXERCISES

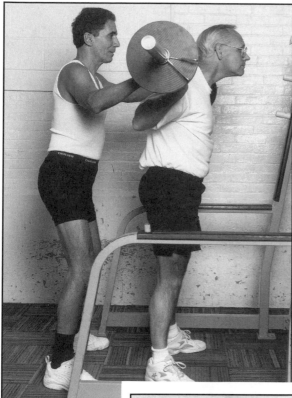

Beginning position.

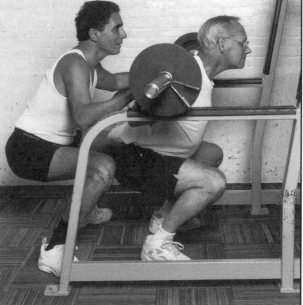

Downward
movement phase.

Machine Leg Press

quadriceps, hamstrings, gluteals

Beginning Position

1. Adjust seat so knees are flexed to 90 degrees or less.
2. Sit with back firmly against seat pad.
3. Place feet flat on foot pad, in line with knees and hips.
4. Grip handles with hands.

Forward Movement Phase

1. Slowly push foot pad forward until knees are almost extended, but not locked.
2. Keep feet, knees, and hips aligned.
3. Exhale throughout pushing phase.

Backward Movement Phase

1. Allow foot pad to slowly return to starting position.
2. Inhale throughout return movement.

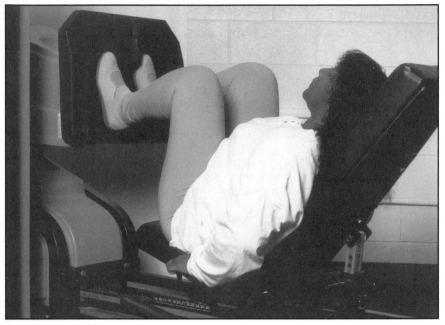

Beginning position.

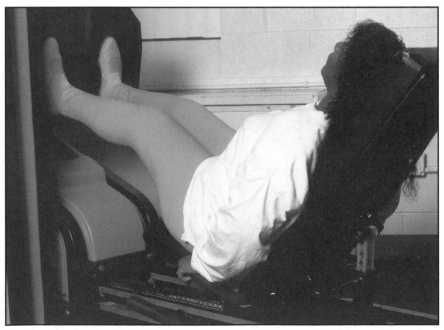

Forward movement phase.

HIPS

Machine Hip Adduction

hip adductors

Beginning Position

1. Sit with back firmly against seat pad.
2. Position knees outside of movement pads and ankles on supports.
3. Adjust movement lever to starting position with legs comfortably apart.
4. Grip handles with hands.

Inward Movement Phase

1. Slowly pull movement pads together.
2. Exhale throughout pulling movement.

Outward Movement Phase

1. Allow pads to slowly return to starting position with legs apart.
2. Inhale throughout return movement.

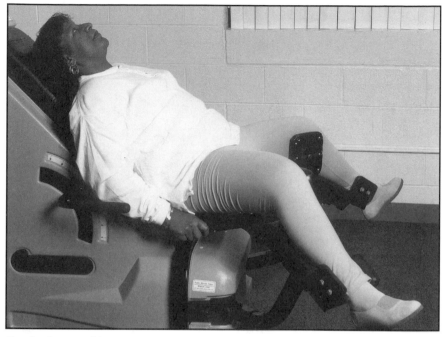

Beginning position.

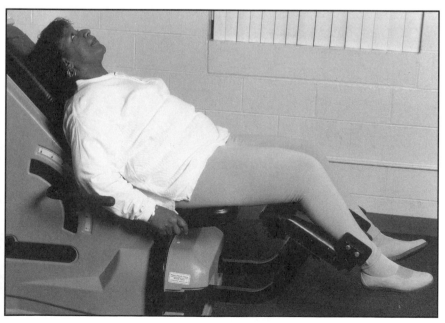

Inward movement phase.

Machine Hip Abduction

hip abductors

Beginning Position

1. Sit with back firmly against seat pad.
2. Position both knees inside of movement pads and ankles on supports with legs together.
3. Grip handles with hands.

Outward Movement Phase

1. Slowly push movement pads apart as far as comfortable.
2. Exhale throughout pushing movement.

Inward Movement Phase

1. Allow movement pads to slowly return to starting position with legs together.
2. Inhale throughout return movement.

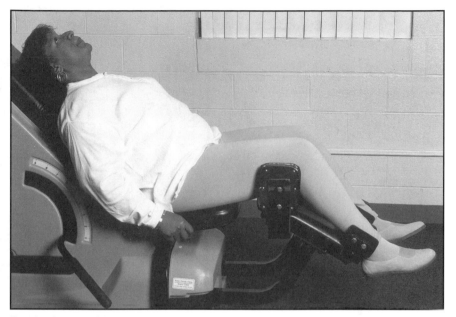

Beginning position.

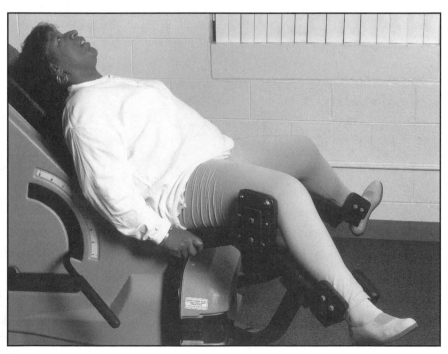

Outward movement phase.

CALVES

Free-Weight Dumbbell Heel Raise

gastrocnemius, soleus

Beginning Position

1. Grasp dumbbells with an overhand grip and stand erect.
2. Position dumbbells with palms facing the outside surfaces of the thighs.
3. Place balls of feet on a *stable,* elevated surface (approximately four inches high), feet hip-width apart and parallel to each other.

Upward Movement Phase

1. Keep head up, eyes fixed straight ahead, shoulders back, back straight, and weight on balls of the feet throughout the upward and downward movement phases of this exercise.
2. Rise up slowly on the toes while keeping torso erect and knees straight.
3. Exhale throughout upward movement.

Downward Movement Phase

1. Lower the heels as far as comfortable while keeping torso erect and knees straight.
2. Inhale throughout lowering movement.

LOWER BODY EXERCISES

Beginning position.

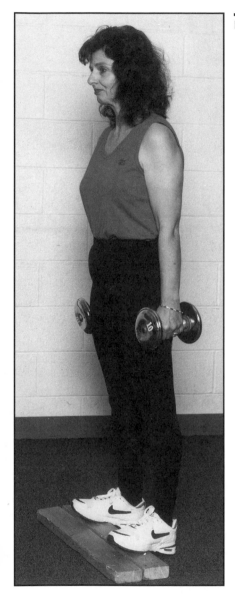

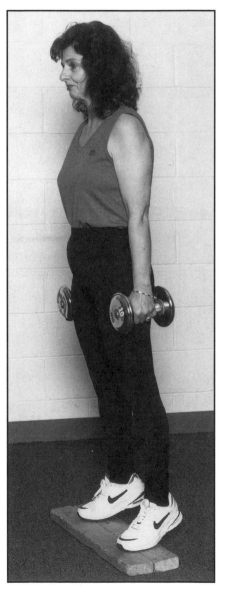

Upward movement phase.

Free-Weight Barbell Heel Raise

gastrocnemius, soleus

Beginning Position

1. Stand erect, position feet shoulder-width apart and grip the bar overhand.
2. Hold bar against thighs with arms straight, head up, and eyes looking ahead. (Another way to perform this exercise is with the bar on shoulders at base of neck. Please note, this variation requires a spotter).
3. Place balls of feet on a *stable,* elevated surface (approximately four inches high), feet hip-width apart and parallel to each other.

Upward Movement Phase

1. Keep head up, eyes fixed straight ahead, shoulders back, back straight, and weight on balls of feet throughout the upward and downward movement phases of this exercise.
2. Slowly rise on toes while keeping torso erect and knees straight.
3. Exhale throughout upward movement.

Downward Movement Phase

1. Lower the heels as far as comfortable while keeping torso erect and knees straight.
2. Inhale throughout lowering movement.

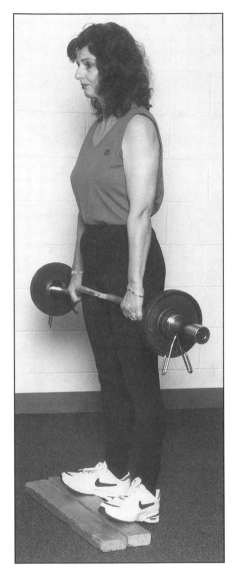

Beginning position.

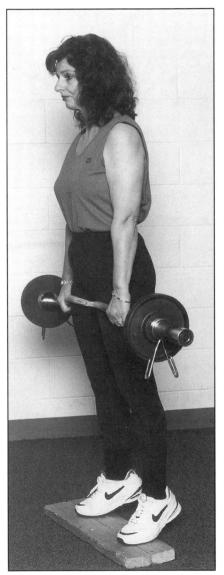

Upward movement phase.

Machine Heel Raise

gastrocnemius, soleus

Beginning Position

1. Position and secure the resistance belt around waist.
2. Stand with balls of feet on rear edge of step.
3. Place hands on support bar.
4. Allow heels to drop below step as far as comfortable.

Upward Movement Phase

1. Slowly rise on toes to lift heels upward as high as possible.
2. Keep knees straight.
3. Exhale throughout upward movement.

Downward Movement Phase

1. Return slowly to starting position, heels below step.
2. Inhale throughout downward movement.

LOWER BODY EXERCISES

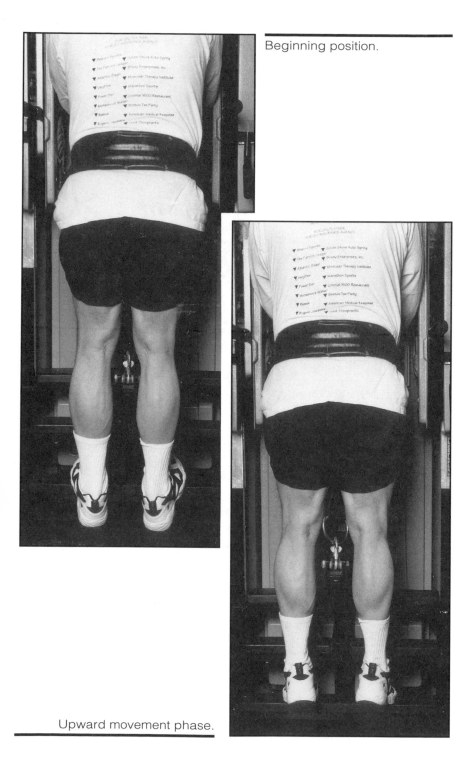

Beginning position.

Upward movement phase.

Midsection Exercises

In this section you will find 4 exercises which address the midsection of the body. These include exercises for strengthening the back and abdominals.

LOW BACK

Machine Back Extension

erector spinae

Beginning Position

1. Sit all the way back on seat and adjust foot pad so knees are slightly higher than hips.
2. Secure seat belt across thighs and hips.
3. Cross arms on chest.
4. Place upper back firmly against pad with trunk flexed forward.

Backward Movement Phase

1. Push upper back against pad until trunk is fully extended.
2. Keep head in line with torso.
3. Exhale throughout extension movement.

Forward Movement Phase

1. Allow the pad to slowly return to starting position.
2. Inhale throughout return movement.

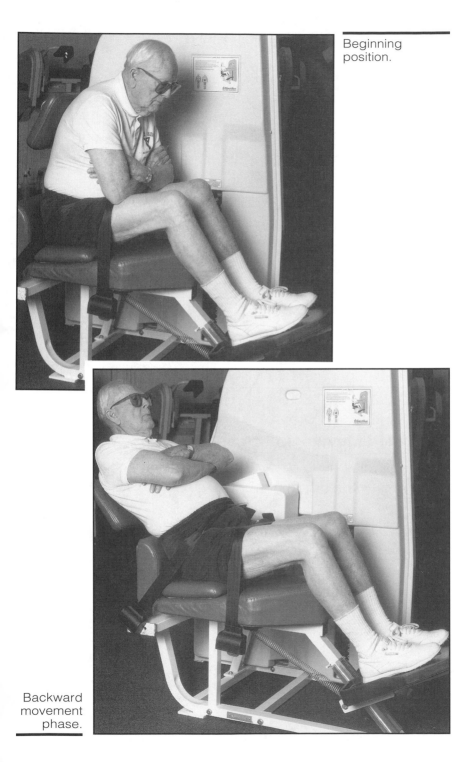

Beginning
position.

Backward
movement
phase.

Machine Abdominal Curl

rectus abdominis

Beginning Position

1. Adjust seat so navel is aligned with machine's axis of rotation.
2. Secure seat belt.
3. Sit with upper back firmly against pad.
4. Place elbows on arm pads and hands on handles.

Forward Movement Phase

1. Slowly pull pad forward until trunk is fully flexed by contracting abdominal muscles (tightening abdominal muscles as tight as you can get them).
2. Keep upper back firmly against pad.
3. Exhale throughout forward movement.

Backward Movement Phase

1. Allow the pad to slowly return to starting position.
2. Inhale throughout return movement.

Beginning position.

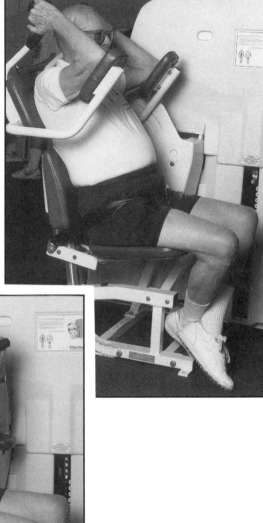

Forward movement phase.

Free-Weight Trunk Curl

rectus abdominis

Beginning Position

1. Lie on back on mat or carpeted floor.
2. Flex knees to 110 degrees, feet flat on the floor.
3. Place hands loosely behind head to maintain neutral neck position.

Upward Movement Phase

1. Slowly raise shoulders about 30 degrees off floor.
2. Exhale throughout upward movement.

Downward Movement Phase

1. Slowly lower shoulders to floor.
2. Inhale throughout lowering movement.

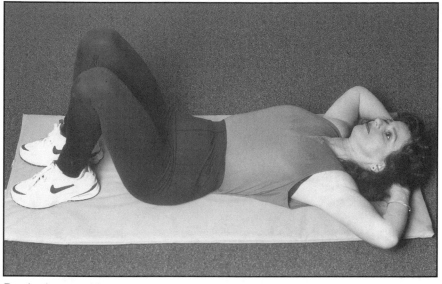

Beginning position.

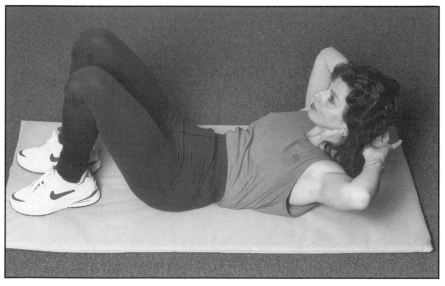

Upward movement phase.

Machine Rotary Torso

rectus abdominis, external obliques, internal obliques

Beginning Position

1. Sit all the way back on seat with torso erect, facing forward.
2. Wrap legs around seat extension.
3. Position right upper arm behind arm pad and left upper arm against arm pad.

Left Movement Phase

1. Turn torso slowly to left, about 45 degrees.
2. Exhale throughout rotation.

Return Movement Phase

1. Allow torso to slowly return to starting position (facing forward).
2. Inhale throughout return movement.
3. Change seat position and arm positions and repeat exercise to right.

Beginning position.

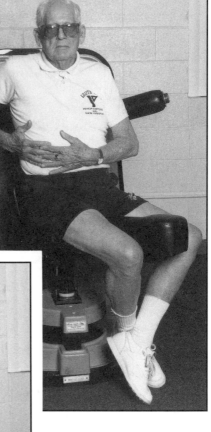

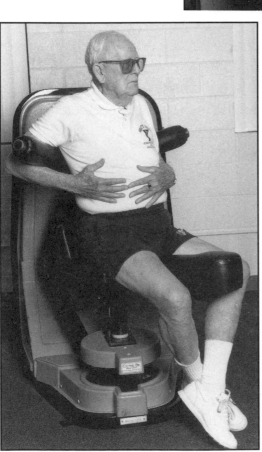

Left movement phase.

Upper Body Exercises

In this section you will find 25 exercises which address the upper body. These include exercises for strengthening the pectorals, upper back, shoulders, and arms.

CHEST

Machine Chest Crossover

pectoralis major, anterior deltoid

Beginning Position

1. Adjust seat so shoulders are in line with machine's axes of rotation and upper arms are parallel to floor.
2. Sit with head, shoulders, and back firmly against seat pad.
3. Position forearms against arm pads and hands on handles.

Forward Movement Phase

1. Pull arm pads slowly together, using arms more than hands.
2. Keep wrists straight.
3. Exhale throughout pulling movement.

Backward Movement Phase

1. Allow arm pads to slowly return to starting position.
2. Inhale throughout return movement.

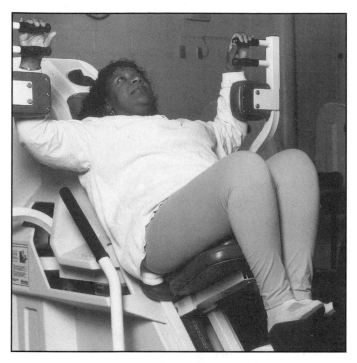

Beginning
position.

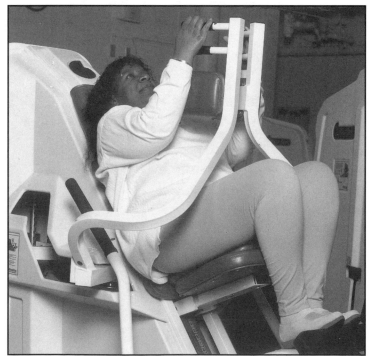

Forward
movement
phase.

Free-Weight Dumbbell Chest Fly

pectoralis major, anterior deltoid

Beginning Position

1. Lie on back on bench with legs straddling bench and knees flexed at 90 degrees, feet flat on the floor.
2. Keep head, shoulders, and buttocks in contact with the bench and feet in contact with the floor throughout exercise.
3. Grasp dumbbells so palms face each other.
4. Push dumbbells in unison to a position over chest with elbows slightly flexed.

Downward Movement Phase

1. Slowly lower dumbbells in unison, keeping elbows slightly flexed and perpendicular to torso.
2. Continue lowering dumbbells until upper arms are parallel to floor.
3. Inhale throughout lowering movement.

Upward Movement Phase

1. Lift dumbbells upward in unison to the starting position (elbows slightly flexed).
2. Exhale throughout upward movement.

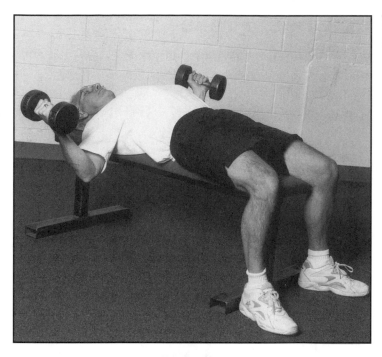

Beginning position.

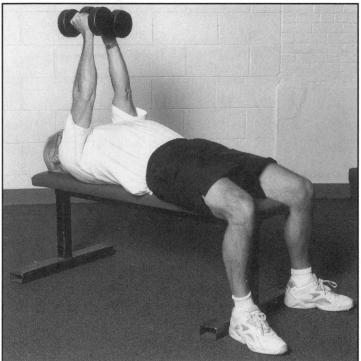

Upward movement phase.

Machine Chest Press

pectoralis major, anterior deltoid, triceps

Beginning Position

1. Adjust seat so handles are right below shoulder level.
2. Sit with head, shoulders, and back against seat pad.
3. Place feet on foot pad and press forward to bring handles into starting position by chest.
4. Grasp handles with fingers and thumbs.
5. Release foot pad slowly.

Forward Movement Phase

1. Push handles forward slowly until arms are fully extended.
2. Keep wrists straight.
3. Exhale throughout pushing movement.

Backward Movement Phase

1. Allow handles to return slowly to the starting position.
2. Inhale throughout the return phase.
3. After completing the final repetition, place feet on foot pad and press forward to hold weightstack, release hand grips, and lower weightstack slowly.

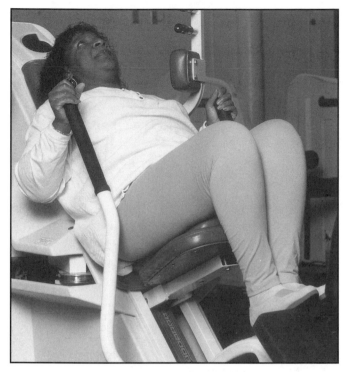

Beginning
position.

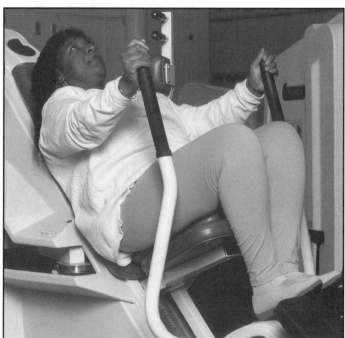

Forward
movement
phase.

Free-Weight Dumbbell Bench Press

pectoralis major, anterior deltoid, triceps

Beginning Position

1. Lie on back with legs straddling bench, knees flexed at 90 degrees, feet flat on floor.
2. Keep head, shoulders, and buttocks in contact with the bench and feet in contact with the floor throughout the exercise.
3. Grasp dumbbells so palms face away and push upward until arms are fully extended above chest.

Downward Movement Phase

1. Slowly lower dumbbells in unison to the outsides of chest.
2. Inhale throughout lowering movement.

Upward Movement Phase

1. Press dumbbells upward in unison until arms are fully extended.
2. Exhale throughout upward movement.

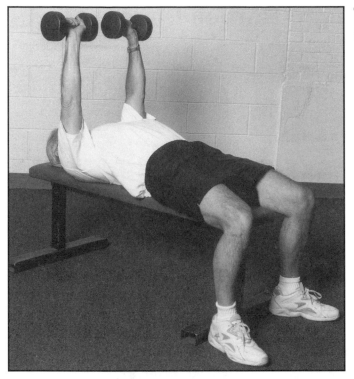

Beginning position.

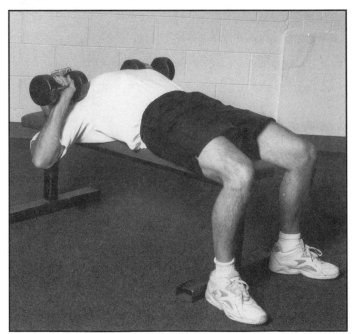

Downward movement phase.

Free-Weight Barbell Bench Press

pectoralis major, anterior deltoid, triceps

Beginning Position

1. Lie on back with legs straddling bench, knees flexed at 90 degrees, feet flat on floor.
2. Keep head, shoulders, and buttocks in contact with the bench and feet in contact with the floor throughout the exercise.
3. Grasp barbell so palms face away and push upward until arms are fully extended above chest.

Downward Movement Phase

1. Slowly and evenly lower bar to nipple area of chest.
2. Inhale throughout the lowering movement.

Upward Movement Phase

1. Press bar upward evenly until arms are fully extended.
2. Exhale throughout pressing movement.

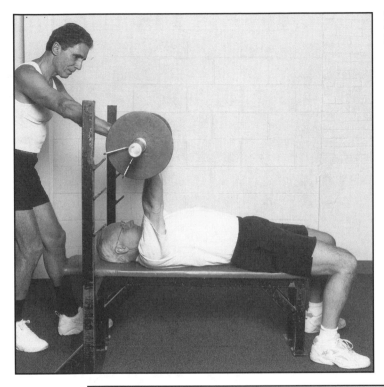

Beginning position.

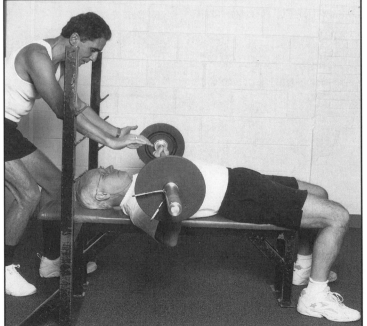

Downward movement phase.

Machine Weight-Assisted Bar-Dip

pectoralis major, triceps

Beginning Position

1. Keep in mind that adding weights makes this exercise easier because they counterbalance your body weight.
2. Climb steps and grasp dip bars with an overhand grip.
3. Place knees on platform and descend until elbows are flexed about 90 degrees.

Upward Movement Phase

1. Slowly push body upward until arms are fully extended.
2. Keep wrists straight.
3. Keep back straight.
4. Exhale throughout pushing movement.

Downward Movement Phase

1. Return slowly to starting position (until elbows are flexed about 90 degrees).
2. Inhale throughout return movement.

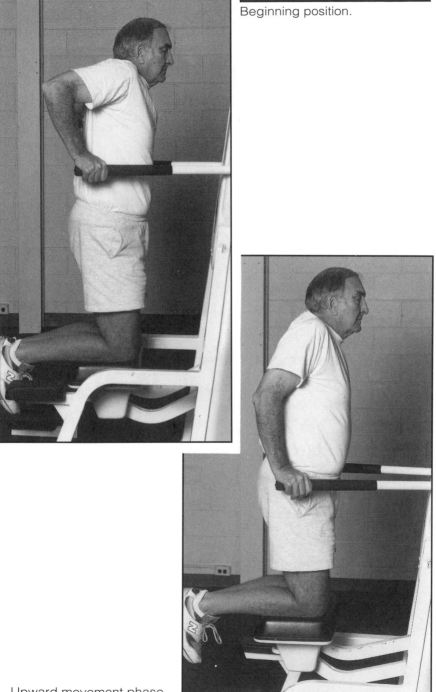

Beginning position.

Upward movement phase.

UPPER BACK

Machine Super-Pullover

latissimus dorsi

Beginning Position

1. Adjust seat so shoulders are in line with machine's axis of rotation.
2. Sit with back firmly against seat pad, seat belt secured.
3. Place feet on foot lever and press forward to bring arm pads into starting position by face.
4. Position arms against arm pads and hands on bar.
5. Release foot pad.

Downward Movement Phase

1. Slowly pull arm pads downward, leading with elbows until bar touches body.
2. Keep wrists straight.
3. Allow back to round slightly during downward movement.
4. Exhale throughout downward movement.

Upward Movement Phase

1. Allow arm pads to slowly return to starting position.
2. Inhale throughout return movement.
3. After completing the final repetition, place feet on foot lever, press forward to hold weightstack; remove arms, and lower weightstack slowly.

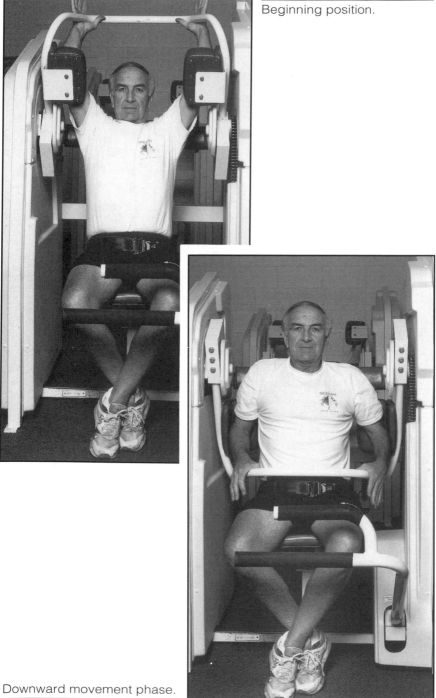

Beginning position.

Downward movement phase.

Free-Weight Dumbbell One-Arm Row

latissimus dorsi, biceps

Beginning Position

1. Grasp dumbbell with right hand and support your weight by placing left hand and knee on the bench, keeping the right leg straight, and right foot flat on floor.
2. Position dumbbell so that palm faces bench, keeping arm straight.
3. Keep back flat throughout exercise.

Upward Movement Phase

1. Slowly pull the dumbbell to the chest.
2. Exhale throughout pulling movement.

Downward Movement Phase

1. Slowly lower dumbbell to starting position.
2. Exhale throughout lowering movement.
3. Repeat exercise from beginning position with left arm.

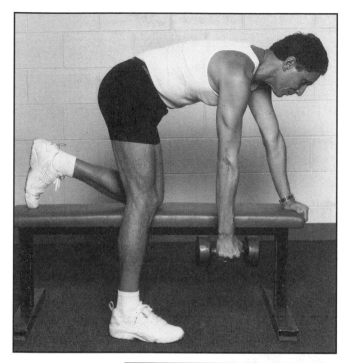

Beginning
position.

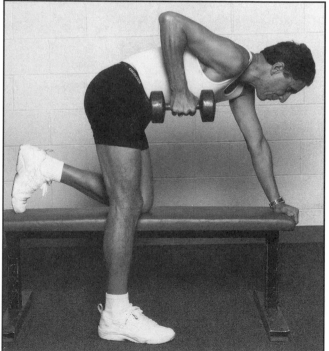

Upward
movement
phase.

Machine Compound Row

latissimus dorsi, biceps

Beginning Position

1. Adjust seat so handles are at shoulder level.
2. Sit with chest against chest pad and torso erect.
3. Place feet flat on floor.
4. Grasp each handle, arms fully extended.

Backward Movement Phase

1. Slowly pull handles back toward chest.
2. Keep wrists straight.
3. Exhale throughout pulling movement.

Forward Movement Phase

1. Allow handles to return slowly until arms are fully extended.
2. Inhale throughout return movement.

Beginning position.

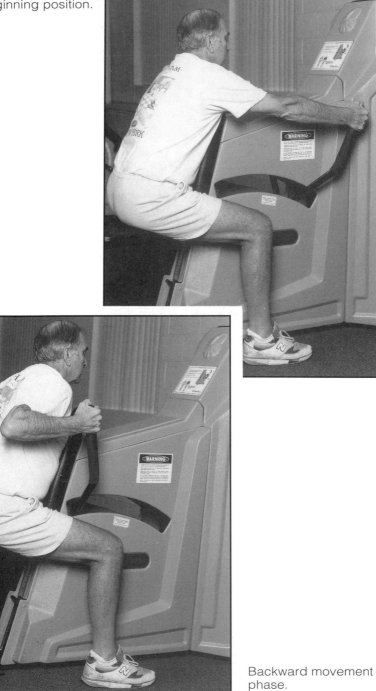

Backward movement
phase.

Machine Lat Pull-Down

latissimus dorsi, biceps

Beginning Position

1. Place knees under restraining pads, keeping upper torso upright.
2. Grip the bar underhand, greater than shoulder-width apart, and arms straight.

Downward Movement Phase

1. Slowly pull bar downward below chin.
2. Exhale throughout pulling movement.

Upward Movement Phase

1. Be prepared for an unexpected upward pull from the bar during the upward movement phase!
2. Allow bar to return slowly until arms are fully extended.
3. Exhale throughout the upward movement.

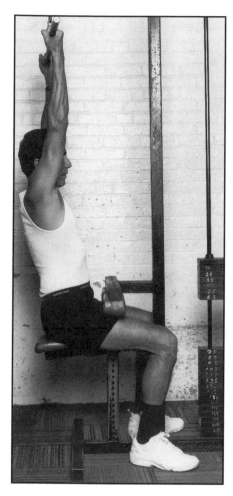

Beginning position.

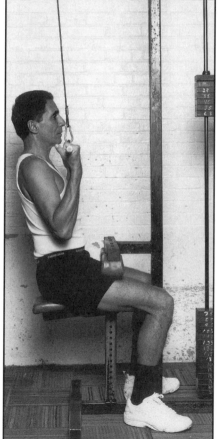

Downward movement phase.

Machine Weight-Assisted Pull-Up

latissimus dorsi, biceps

Beginning Position

1. Keep in mind that adding weights makes this exercise easier because they counterbalance your body weight.
2. Climb steps and grasp chin bar with an underhand grip.
3. Place knees on platform and descend until arms are fully extended.

Upward Movement Phase

1. Pull body upward until chin is above chin bar.
2. Keep wrists straight.
3. Keep back straight.
4. Exhale throughout pulling movement.

Downward Movement Phase

1. Slowly return to starting position (until arms are fully extended).
2. Inhale throughout return movement.

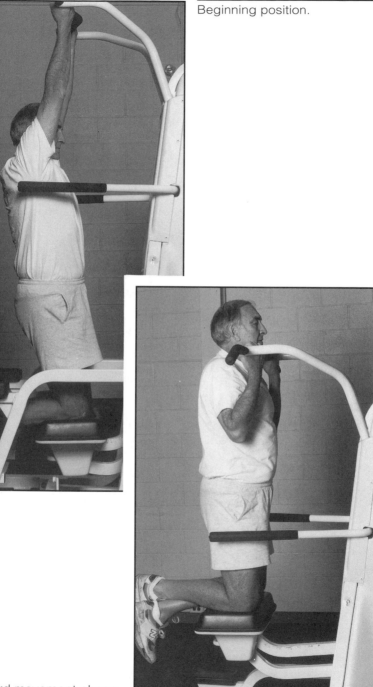

Beginning position.

Upward movement phase.

SHOULDERS

Free-Weight Dumbbell Seated Press

deltoids, triceps

Beginning Position

1. Sit with legs straddling bench and feet in contact with floor at all times.
2. Grasp dumbbells with palms turned forward, positioned at shoulder height.
3. If you're using an upright or adjustable bench, keep head and entire back in contact with it.

Upward Movement Phase

1. Slowly push dumbbells upward in unison until arms are fully extended over the shoulders.
2. Exhale throughout pushing movement.

Downward Movement Phase

1. Slowly lower dumbbells in unison to shoulder level.
2. Inhale throughout lowering movement.

Beginning position.

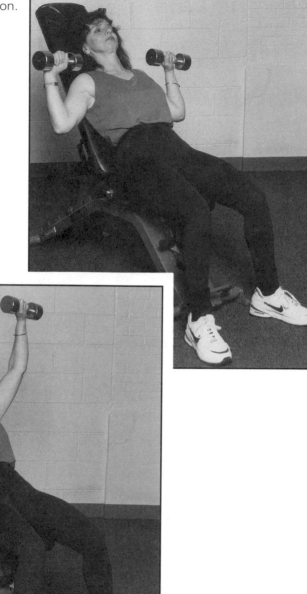

Upward movement phase.

Machine Lateral Raise

deltoids

Beginning Position

1. Adjust seat so shoulders are in line with machine's axis of rotation.
2. Sit with head, shoulders, and back firmly against seat pad.
3. Position arms against arm pads and hands on handles, with arms close to sides.

Upward Movement Phase

1. Slowly lift arm pads upward, using arms more than hands.
2. Keep wrists straight.
3. Stop upward movement when arms are parallel to floor.
4. Exhale throughout lifting movement.

Downward Movement Phase

1. Allow pads to slowly return to starting position.
2. Inhale throughout lowering movement.

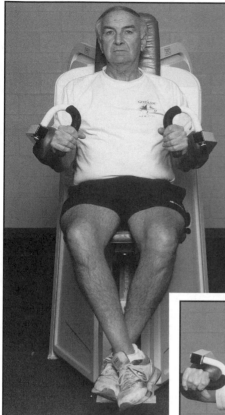

Beginning position.

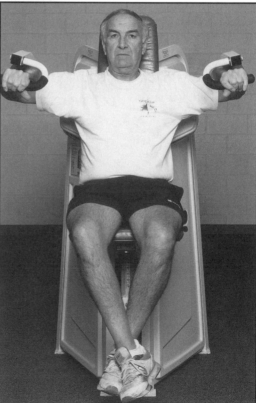

Upward movement phase.

Free-Weight Dumbbell Lateral Raise

deltoids

Beginning Position

1. Grasp dumbbells with palms facing the outside of thighs and elbows slightly flexed.
2. Stand erect with feet hip-width apart.

Upward Movement Phase

1. Slowly lift dumbbells upward in unison until level with shoulders, arms parallel to floor.
2. Exhale throughout the upward movement.

Downward Movement Phase

1. Slowly lower dumbbells in unison to starting position.
2. Inhale throughout lowering movement.

UPPER BODY EXERCISES

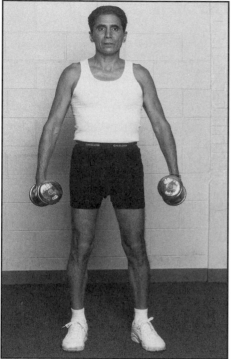

Beginning position.

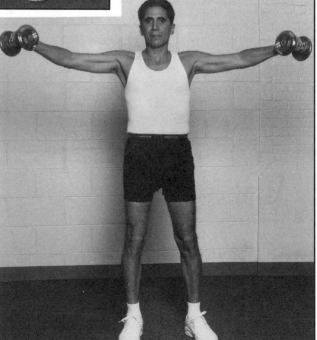

Upward move-
ment phase.

Free-Weight Dumbbell Shrug

upper trapezius

Beginning Position

1. Grasp dumbbells with overhand grip, arms at sides and fully extended. Keep arms straight throughout the exercise.
2. Stand erect with feet hip-width apart.

Upward Movement Phase

1. Elevate (shrug) the shoulders in unison toward the ears as high as possible.
2. Exhale throughout shrugging movement.

Downward Movement Phase

1. Slowly lower dumbbells in unison to starting position.
2. Exhale throughout lowering movement.

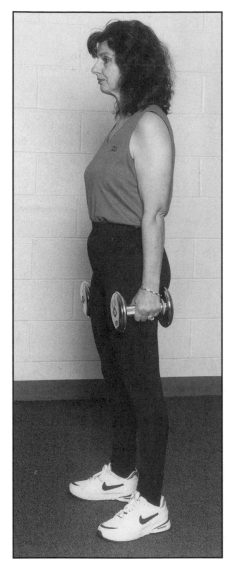

Beginning position.

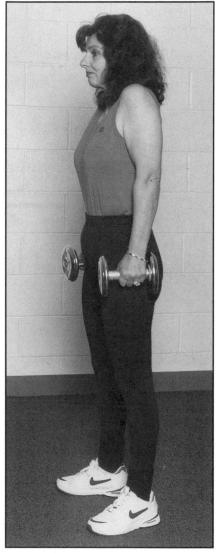

Upward movement phase.

Free-Weight Barbell Shrug

upper trapezius

Beginning Position

1. Grasp barbell with an overhand grip, arms at sides and fully extended. Keep arms straight throughout the exercise.
2. Stand erect with feet hip-width apart.

Upward Movement Phase

1. Elevate (shrug) the shoulders toward the ears as high as possible.
2. Exhale throughout shrugging movement.

Downward Movement Phase

1. Slowly lower barbell to starting position.
2. Inhale throughout lowering movement.

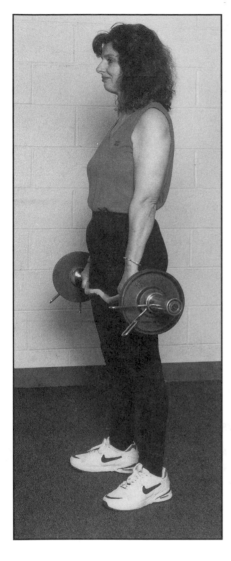

Beginning position.

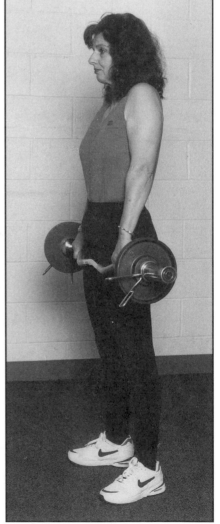

Upward movement phase.

ARMS

Machine Biceps Curl

biceps

Beginning Position

1. Adjust seat so elbows are in line with machine's axis of rotation and upper arms are parallel to floor.
2. Grasp handles with underhand grip, elbows slightly flexed.
3. Sit with chest against chest pad, torso erect.

Upward Movement Phase

1. Slowly curl handles upward until elbows are fully flexed.
2. Keep wrists straight.
3. Exhale throughout lifting movement.

Downward Movement Phase

1. Allow handles to return slowly to starting position.
2. Inhale throughout lowering movement.

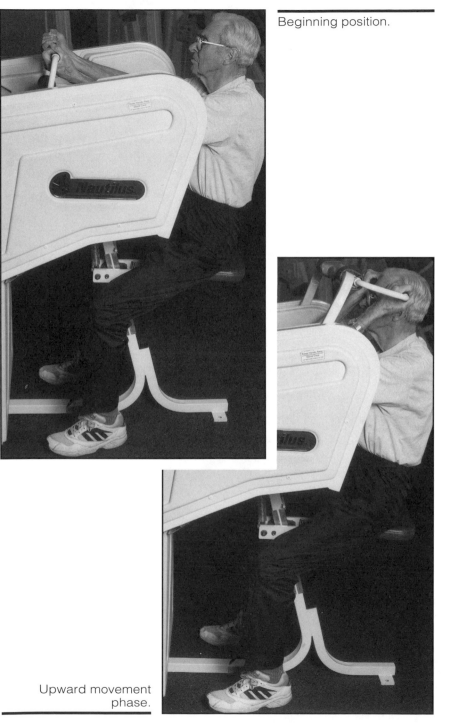

Beginning position.

Upward movement
phase.

Free-Weight Dumbbell Curl

biceps

Beginning Position

1. Grasp dumbbells with palms facing outsides of thighs, and arms straight. Ensure that upper arms remain perpendicular to floor and against sides throughout this exercise.
2. Stand erect with feet about hip-width apart and parallel to each other.

Upward Movement Phase

1. Curl dumbbells upward in unison toward shoulders by rotating wrists until palms face the chest.
2. Exhale throughout upward movement.

Downward Movement Phase

1. Slowly lower dumbbells in unison to starting position.
2. Inhale throughout lowering movement.

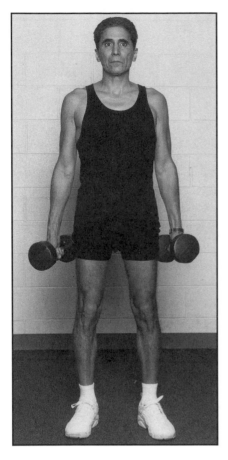

Beginning position.

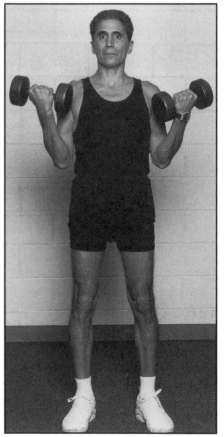

Upward movement phase.

Free-Weight Dumbbell Concentration Curl

biceps

Beginning Position

1. Sit on bench, grasp dumbbell in left hand with right arm braced against left thigh, feet shoulder-width apart, and upper body leaning slightly forward. Upper arm should remain firmly braced against thigh throughout the exercise.
2. Begin with arm straight and palm facing forward.

Upward Movement Phase

1. Curl dumbbell toward chin.
2. Exhale throughout curling movement.

Downward Movement Phase

1. Slowly lower dumbbell back to starting position.
2. Inhale throughout lowering movement.
3. Repeat from beginning position with left arm.

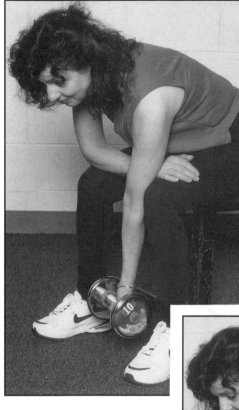

Beginning position.

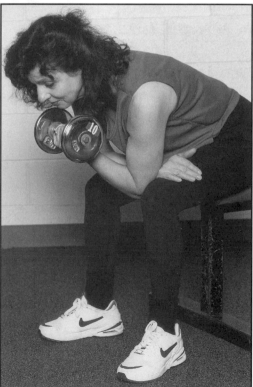

Upward movement phase.

Free-Weight Barbell Curl

biceps

Beginning Position

1. Grasp bar with underhand grip, with upper arms against sides. Ensure that upper arms remain perpendicular to floor and against sides throughout this exercise.
2. Stand erect with feet about hip-width apart and parallel to each other.

Upward Movement Phase

1. Slowly curl barbell upward toward shoulders.
2. Exhale throughout curling movement.

Downward Movement Phase

1. Slowly lower barbell until arms are fully extended.
2. Inhale throughout lowering movement.

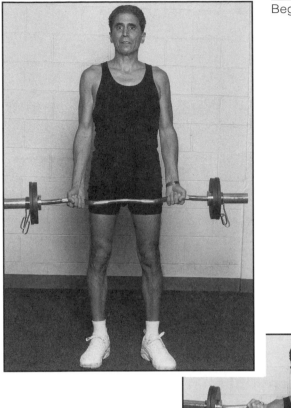

Beginning position.

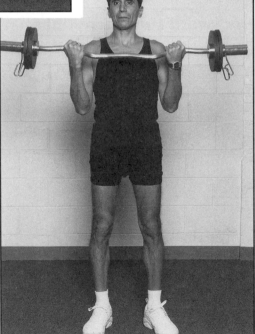

Upward movement phase.

Machine Triceps Extension

triceps

Beginning Position

1. Adjust seat so elbows are in line with machine's axis of rotation.
2. Sit with back firmly against seat pad.
3. Place sides of hands against hand pads and allow pads to move close to face.

Forward Movement Phase

1. Slowly push hand pads forward until arms are fully extended.
2. Keep wrists straight.
3. Exhale throughout forward movement.

Backward Movement Phase

1. Allow pads to return slowly to the starting position.
2. Inhale throughout return movement.
3. After the final repetition, stand to remove hands from hand pads and exit seat.

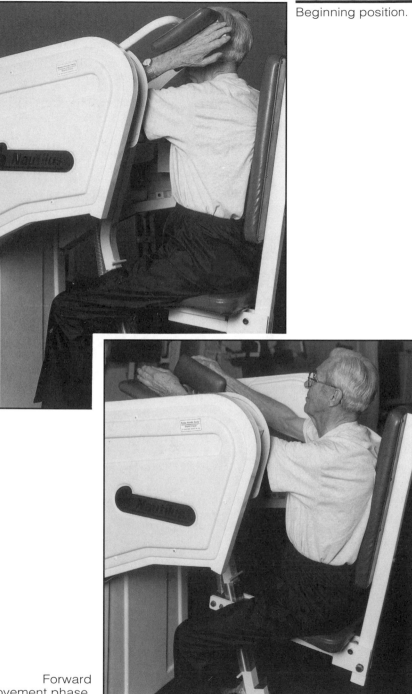

Beginning position.

Forward
movement phase.

Free-Weight Dumbbell Overhead Triceps Extension

triceps

Beginning Position

1. Grasp one dumbbell with both hands and stand erect with feet about hip-width apart.
2. Lift dumbbell upward until arms are fully extended, directly above head. Keep upper arms perpendicular to floor throughout exercise.

Downward Movement Phase

1. Slowly lower dumbbell toward base of neck.
2. Exhale throughout lowering movement.

Upward Movement Phase

1. Lift dumbbell upward slowly until arms are fully extended.
2. Inhale throughout lifting movement.

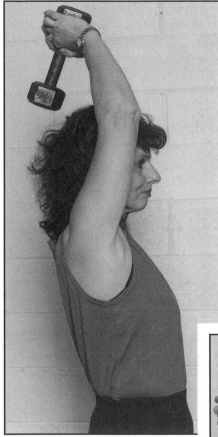

Beginning position.

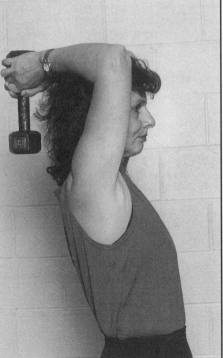

Downward movement phase.

Machine Triceps Press-Down

triceps

Beginning Position

1. Stand erect with feet hip-width apart and knees slightly flexed.
2. Grasp bar with overhand grip.
3. Push bar down until upper arms are perpendicular with floor and touching sides.

Downward Movement Phase

1. Push bar downward until arms are fully extended.
2. Exhale throughout pushing movement.

Upward Movement Phase

1. Be prepared for an unexpected upward pull from the bar during the upward movement phase!
2. Return bar slowly to starting position.
3. Inhale throughout upward movement.

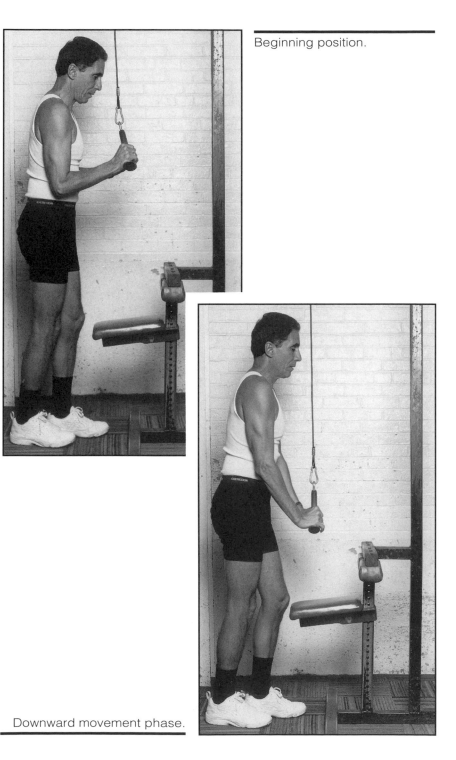

Beginning position.

Downward movement phase.

NECK

Machine Neck Flexion

neck flexors

Beginning Position

1. Adjust seat so face will fit comfortably against head pad, nose parallel to crossbar.
2. Adjust torso pad for erect posture.
3. Place forehead and cheeks against head pad, head angled slightly backward.
4. Grip handles.

Forward Movement Phase

1. Push head pad forward slowly until the neck is fully flexed.
2. Keep torso straight.
3. Exhale throughout forward movement.

Backward Movement Phase

1. Allow head pad to return slowly to starting position, with head angled slightly backward.
2. Inhale throughout return movement.

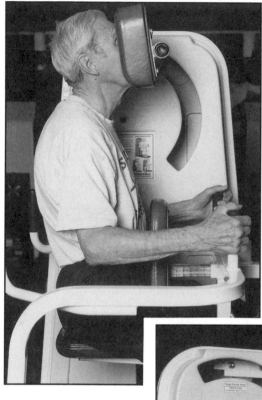

Beginning position.

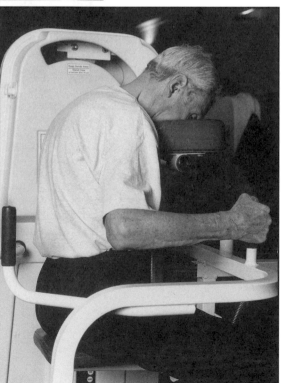

Forward movement phase.

Machine Neck Extension

neck extensors

Beginning Position

1. Adjust seat so back of head fits comfortably in head pad.
2. Adjust torso pad for an erect posture.
3. Place back of head against head pad with head angled slightly forward.
4. Grip handles.

Backward Movement Phase

1. Push head pad backward slowly until neck is comfortably extended.
2. Keep torso straight.
3. Exhale throughout backward movement.

Forward Movement Phase

1. Allow head pad to slowly return to starting position, with head angled slightly forward.
2. Inhale throughout return movement.

▶ **Note:** Because the neck area is potentially difficult to train correctly and safely, we have not included these exercises in the sample workouts. However, we encourage you to consider exercising these important muscles regularly with instruction from your personal trainer or qualified fitness professional.

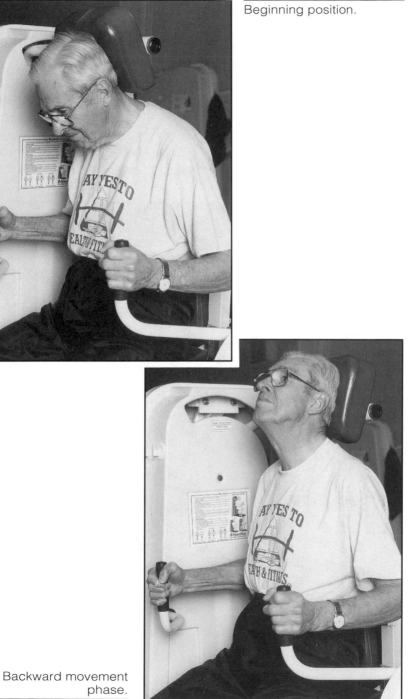

Beginning position.

Backward movement phase.

Additional Machine Exercises

Although your forearm muscles are involved in all gripping exercises (e.g., holding dumbbells, barbells, chinning bars, and so on), some facilities have specially designed forearm machines that target these muscles. For example, the Nautilus super-forearm machine features five separate exercises for the various forearm muscles (see figure below). If you have access to this machine, be sure to consult an instructor to ensure that you perform the forearm exercises properly.

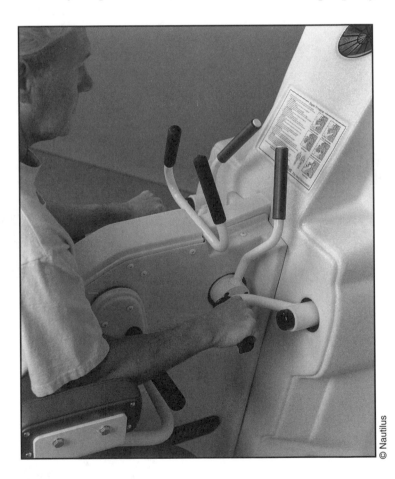

© Nautilus

chapter

6

Building an Effective Training Program

Your key to stronger muscles is a progressive training system that gradually increases exercise resistance. The primary goal of the training programs in this text is to challenge the target muscles during each set of an exercise. That is, you should use a weightload that you are able to lift for about 30 to 90 seconds with good form. A resistance you cannot lift for at least 30 seconds is too heavy and may increase your risk of injury. A resistance you can lift more than 90 seconds is probably too light and may decrease your training benefits.

Let's assume that you can perform 10 controlled leg extensions with 50 pounds in about 60 seconds. This is an ideal exercise resistance for you. As your thigh muscles become stronger, however, you will perform more repetitions with this weightload. To become even stronger, you must now add a little more resistance to more effectively **overload** these muscles.

Overload—Loading the muscles with progressively more resistance than they have previously encountered as they become stronger.

In this chapter, we'll present our research-based guidelines for safe and successful strength

129

training. To address the key components of your strength-training program, we'll make recommendations in the following areas:

- Training Principles
- Technique Factors
- Program Factors

Training Principles

Training Principles include

- exercise selection and order,
- training frequency,
- exercise sets,
- exercise resistance,
- exercise repetitions,
- training progression, and
- training effort.

Exercise Selection and Order

Many people select certain exercises because they are more popular, more convenient, or more satisfying to perform than others. For example, most strength-training programs feature bench presses for upper body development. It is true that bench presses strengthen the chest muscles and triceps. However, if you do not give equal attention to the *opposing muscles* in your upper back and biceps, you may develop a *strength imbalance* between your upper body's pushing and pulling muscles. This may lead to poor posture and susceptibility to joint injuries.

Opposing muscles—Muscles on opposite sides of a joint, one that produces joint flexion and the other that produces joint extension.

Strength imbalance—Developing disproportionate strength on one side of a joint by emphasizing one muscle over its opposite.

▶ **Recommendation:** Train all your major muscle groups to develop balanced strength throughout your muscular system.

Also, you may begin your machine workout with leg extensions for the front-of-thigh muscles followed by leg curls for the back-of-thigh muscles. This works your larger muscles while you are fresh and ensures balanced training for your legs.

▶ **Recommendation:** Train opposing muscle groups in pairs.

After training your legs, you may do exercises for your upper body muscles, including the chest, upper back, and shoulders. Sample machine exercises for these muscles are the chest crossover for the chest, super-pullover for the upper back, and lateral raise for the shoulders. Sample free-weight exercises are the dumbbell chest fly for the chest, dumbbell one-arm row for the upper back, and dumbbell lateral raise for the shoulders.

Next in the training order are your upper arm muscles. For example, you may do a set of biceps curls on the biceps machine and a set of triceps extensions on the triceps machine to address these muscles in a balanced manner. For free weights, you may choose dumbbell curls and dumbbell overhead triceps extensions.

The last muscles in your training sequence are those of the midsection. Because these muscles help to stabilize your spinal column as you perform most exercises, you don't want to fatigue them until the end of the workout. You may use the low back machine and the abdominal machine for your midsection muscles. If you are doing the free-weight program, this is the logical place in your workout for trunk curls.

Once you master the basic training program, you may add exercises for your inner and outer thighs, the sides of your midsection, your lower legs, and perhaps your forearms and neck. Table 6.1 presents sample machine and free-weight exercises for each of the major muscle groups.

Of course, you do not always have to train in the recommended exercise sequence. For example, you may occasionally

Table 6.1

SUGGESTED EXERCISES FOR MAJOR MUSCLE GROUPS

Muscle group	Machine exercise	Free-weight exercise
Front-of-thigh (Quadriceps)	Leg extension	Dumbbell squat or barbell squat
Back-of-thigh (Hamstrings)	Leg curl	Dumbbell squat or barbell squat
Inner thigh (Hip adductors)	Hip adduction	
Outer thigh (Hip abductors)	Hip abduction	
Lower leg (Gastrocnemius)	Heel raise	Dumbbell heel raise
Chest (Pectoralis major)	Chest crossover	Dumbbell bench press or barbell bench press
Upper back (Latissimus dorsi)	Super-pullover	Dumbbell one-arm row
Shoulders (Deltoids)	Lateral raise	Dumbbell seated press
Front-of-arm (Biceps)	Biceps curl	Dumbbell biceps curl
Back-of-arm (Triceps)	Triceps extension	Dumbbell overhead extension
Low back (Erector spinae)	Back extension	
Abdominals (Rectus abdominis)	Abdominal curl	Trunk curl
Sides (External and internal obliques)	Rotary torso	Twisting trunk curl
Front neck (Neck flexors)	Neck flexion	
Rear neck (Neck extensors)	Neck extension	
Forearms (Wrist flexors and extensors)	Forearm	

want to work your weaker muscle groups first while you are fresh. Keep in mind though, that when you vary the exercise order, that the number of repetitions you can perform will change accordingly. That is, you should be able to perform more repetitions with your weaker muscles because you are less fatigued in the early stages of your workout.

It may be that lack of time or equipment may prevent you from doing all the recommended exercises. If this is the case, you may elect to do a shorter strength-training program, using four machine or free-weight exercises that involve most of your major muscle groups. As shown in table 6.2, this approach includes one exercise for your legs, one for your upper body pushing muscles, one for your upper body pulling muscles, and one for your midsection muscles. Whether you do many or few exercises, be sure to train in a "balanced" manner.

For Lower Strength Levels

You may find that the four-exercise program presented in table 6.2 is sufficient for your first few weeks of strength training.

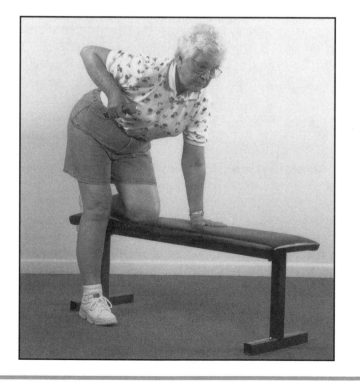

Table 6.2

SAMPLE ABBREVIATED EXERCISE PROGRAM

Muscle group	Free-weight exercise	Machine exercise
Front-and-back-of-thigh, buttocks	Dumbbell squat	Leg press
Chest, shoulders, back-of-arms	Dumbbell/barbell bench press	Chest press
Upper back, shoulders, front-of-arms	Dumbbell one-arm row	Compound row
Midsection	Trunk curl	Abdominal curl

Training Frequency

Regular strength training progressively stresses your muscles and produces some degree of *tissue microtrauma*. Following each training session the exercised tissues rebuild and remodel themselves, resulting in larger and stronger muscles. These tissue-building processes typically take 48 to 72 hours. Although your training frequency may vary, most people make consistent strength improvements with two or three exercise sessions per week.

Tissue microtrauma—Temporary weakening of muscle cells that stimulates tissue-building processes and strength development.

▶ **Recommendation:** You should do strength training two or three nonconsecutive days per week.

An every-other-day program of strength training ensures consistency and produces excellent results. But two strength workouts a week produces almost as much muscle development as three strength workouts a week. As shown in figure 6.1, adults and seniors who trained twice a week added about 88 percent as much lean (muscle) weight as those who trained three times a week.

Based on these studies, we recommend two or three strength-training sessions a week. Although your rate of muscle development may be slightly greater with three workouts a week, a

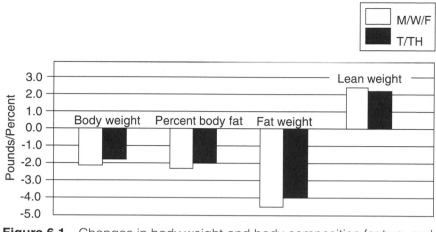

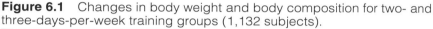

Figure 6.1 Changes in body weight and body composition for two- and three-days-per-week training groups (1,132 subjects).

two-day-a-week training program also produces excellent results.

Actually, your training consistency is just as important as your exercise frequency. Missing scheduled training sessions is unproductive, and working your muscles two days in a row is counterproductive. Thus, we encourage you to establish a regular strength-training workout schedule that is compatible with your lifestyle.

Exercise Sets

An exercise set refers to a group of consecutive repetitions that you perform in a given exercise. For example, if you pick up the dumbbells and do 10 biceps curls and then return the dumbbells to the floor, you have completed one set of 10 repetitions. If you take a rest, then repeat this procedure, you have completed two sets of 10 repetitions.

▶ **Recommendation:** Begin your strength-training program with one set of each exercise.

One set of an exercise is the minimum requirement for strength improvement, and single-set strength training is an efficient and effective means for muscle development. One research study on upper body strength gains—measured by increases in repetitions performed—showed similar results among groups of participants who did one, two, or three sets of chin-ups and bar-dips over a 10-week training period (see figure 6.2).

A University of Florida study compared lower body strength gains—measured by percentage increase in the weightload lifted—for participants who performed one or three sets of leg extensions and leg curls. As illustrated in figure 6.3, both training groups made almost equal gains in lower body strength during the 14-week training period.

▶ **Recommendation:** Although single-set strength training produces excellent results, as you become more

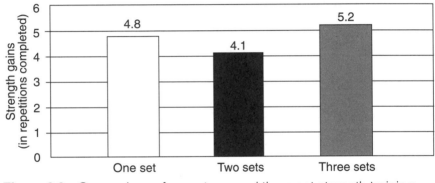

Figure 6.2 Comparison of one-, two-, and three-set strength training (77 subjects).

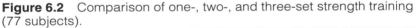

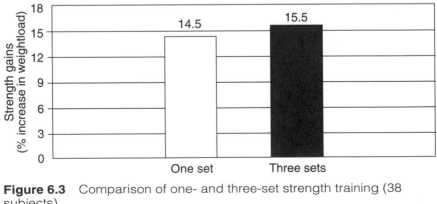

Figure 6.3 Comparison of one- and three-set strength training (38 subjects).

advanced you may want to add a second or third set to stimulate more muscle development.

When performing two or more sets of the same exercise, you should allow yourself to recover for about two minutes between sets. This is sufficient time to rest your muscles and restore about 95 percent of your **anaerobic energy** supply.

You may do multiple exercise sets with the same resistance, such as completing three sets of 10 leg extensions, using 50 pounds for each set. You may also do multiple-set training with increasing weightloads, such as a set of 10 leg extensions with 30 pounds, a second set of 10 leg extensions with 40 pounds, and a third set of 10 leg extensions with 50 pounds. This training method provides a warm-up process prior to your heaviest training set. Another training alternative is the pyramid approach, which involves using heavier resistance and fewer repetitions in successive sets. For example, you may do 10 leg extensions with 50 pounds, 8 leg extensions with 60 pounds, and 6 repetitions with 70 pounds.

Anaerobic energy system— Energy for high-effort exercise that can be performed less than 90 seconds due to muscular fatigue.

▶ **Recommendation:** As a general training guideline, we recommend beginning with one set of each exercise, gradually adding more sets if you desire. If you do multiple exercise sets, be sure to rest at least two minutes between each set.

Exercise Resistance

For decades, the overload principle has been the basic premise of strength training. Overload means using progressively heavier resistance to work your muscles harder and stimulate further strength development. For example, if you presently are completing 10 bench presses with 100 pounds, you could experience an overload by simply increasing the resistance to 102.5 pounds and doing as many repetitions as you can with this slightly heavier weightload.

It is possible to apply the overload principle by doing low repetitions with relatively heavy weightloads or by doing high repetitions with relatively light weightloads. Using very heavy resistance, however, may increase injury potential and using light resistance may decrease the strength-building stimulus. Most people can complete 8 to 12 repetitions with approximately 75 percent of their maximum resistance (see chapter 2). This is a safe and productive workload that stimulates muscle development without overstressing your joint structures.

When performed at a moderate movement speed (about six seconds per repetition), 8 to 12 repetitions with 75 percent of your maximum resistance requires about 50 to 70 seconds of high-effort exercise. This work effort activates the anaerobic energy system and provides excellent strength gains for most individuals. There is, however, a range of resistances that are effective for muscle development. Generally speaking, you may create a strength-building effect by training between 60 and 90 percent of your maximum resistance.

In summary, training with 75 percent of your maximum resistance provides a high strength-building stimulus and presents a low injury risk. Yet, while this is a standard training procedure, you should periodically train with slightly lower and slightly higher percentages of your maximum resistance. These variations offer welcomed changes in your training, creating both physical and mental benefits.

▶ **Recommendation:** For most training purposes, you should use a weightload you can lift for 8 to 12 repetitions, which is about 75 percent of your maximum resistance.

Exercise Repetitions

You should perform exercise repetitions in a controlled manner that maximizes muscle tension and minimizes movement momentum. Remember, at six seconds per repetition (two-second lifting phase and four-second lowering phase), training with 8 to 12 repetitions requires approximately 50 to 70 seconds of high-effort anaerobic exercise.

In a study by one of the authors (Westcott), 141 subjects were tested to determine how many repetitions they could complete with 75 percent of their maximum resistance. As illustrated in figure 6.4, the majority of participants experienced muscle fatigue within 8 to 12 repetitions.

▶ **Recommendation:** In general, you should perform 8 to 12 repetitions in each exercise set. However, you may periodically perform fewer repetitions with higher resistance and more repetitions with lower resistance, as training variety enhances your strength development.

Although you should experience excellent strength gains performing 8 to 12 repetitions per set, you may systematically change the repetition protocol. For example, during your first training month, you may complete more than 12 repetitions with a lighter resistance as your muscles become accustomed to strength training. During the second training month, you may perform 8 to 12 repetitions with a moderate resistance, and during the third training month, you may do fewer than 8 repetitions with a heavier resistance if you so desire. After a month of higher-resistance training, however, you should return to moderate weightloads (8 to 12 repetitions per set) to reduce the risk of overtraining.

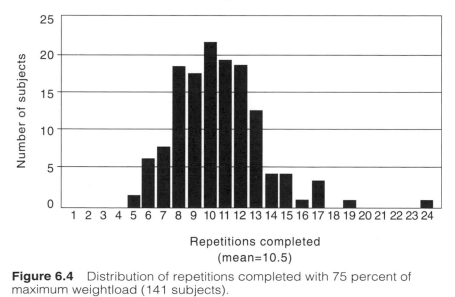

Repetitions completed
(mean=10.5)

Figure 6.4 Distribution of repetitions completed with 75 percent of maximum weightload (141 subjects).

Developing the most productive training protocol may take some experimentation. Although you may periodically change the number of repetitions, you should always work within your anaerobic energy system (approximately 30 to 90 seconds). That is, you should typically do no fewer than 5 repetitions per set and no more than 15 repetitions per set.

Training Progression

As your muscles become stronger, you will be able to do more repetitions with the same exercise resistance. Adding repetitions is productive up to a point. But as the number of repetitions increases , the strength-building stimulus is somewhat diminished. You should, therefore, establish a procedure for gradually increasing your training weightloads.

> ▶ **Recommendation:** Based on the standard training protocol, you should raise your exercise resistance about 2.5 pounds whenever you complete 12 repetitions with proper form in two consecutive workout sessions.

Our experience indicates that a 2.5-pound weightload increase is a safe and productive training progression. For example, if you complete 12 leg presses with 100 pounds during two successive workouts you should use 102.5 pounds your next training session. The 2.5-pound greater resistance should slightly increase your training stimulus and slightly decrease your exercise repetitions. Then when you can complete 12 leg presses with 102.5 pounds, increase the weightload to 105 pounds, and so on.

This procedure—first increasing the repetitions then increasing the resistance—is known as a *double progressive program*. It is a conservative system that reduces the risk of doing too much too soon and consequently experiencing an overtraining injury. Of course, you may apply the double progressive program to other training protocols. For example, if you are doing 12 to 15 repeti-

Double progressive program— A method for systematically increasing the strength-building stimulus by first increasing the repetitions and then increasing the resistance.

For Lower Strength Levels

Stay with the same weightload until you complete 12 repetitions in two consecutive workouts.

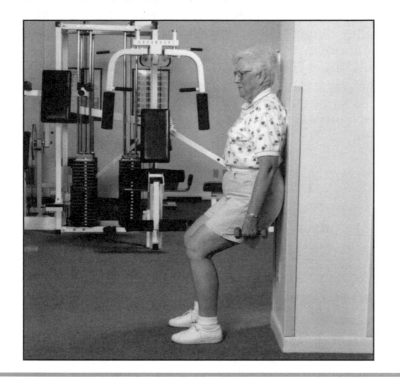

tions per set, you should add 2.5 pounds upon completing 15 repetitions during two consecutive workout sessions.

Training Effort

Exercise physiologists agree that strength development is enhanced by training at a high level of muscle effort. Basically, you'll get the best results when your exercise intensity is high enough to fatigue the target muscles. For most practical purposes, performing one set of 8 to 12 controlled repetitions with 75 percent of your maximum resistance provides sufficient training intensity. As you gain strength fitness, however, you may want to increase your exercise effort.

▶ **Recommendation:** You may increase your training effort by doing more sets of a given exercise or by doing more exercises for a given muscle group.

For example, you may perform a set of leg extensions, rest two minutes, and complete another set of leg extensions. As a more time-efficient alternative, you may perform a set of leg extensions followed closely by a set of leg presses. Both of these exercises target your quadriceps muscles but involve different movement patterns to provide additional training stimulus. Of course, you should only do these advanced training procedures if you want to put greater effort into your exercise program.

Technique Factors

Technique factors include

- movement speed,
- movement range, and
- exercise breathing.

Movement Speed

Movement speed refers to the time required to perform each exercise repetition. This includes the total time you use to lift and lower the weightload (note that lift refers to the direction of the weight stack, barbell, or dumbbell, regardless of your movement pattern). Slower movement speeds involve more muscle tension and less momentum, which should increase your training stimulus and decrease your injury risk. But it is difficult to determine an ideal movement speed for performing strength-training exercises.

In a recent study, the effects of 4-, 6-, 8-, and 14-second repetitions on strength development were compared in 198 men and women (see table 6.3). All four exercise groups made excellent strength gains over an eight-week training period. That is, repetition speeds between 4 and 14 seconds were all effective for improving strength across 13 major muscle groups.

Table 6.3

MOVEMENT SPEED AND STRENGTH IMPROVEMENT

Training protocol (8 weeks)	Reps per set	Time per set (in seconds)	Mean wt. increase (13 Nautilus machines in pounds)
A. 4 sec./rep	10	40	+22
B. 6 sec./rep	10	60	+22
C. 8 sec./rep	10	80	+23
D. 14 sec./rep	5	70	+27

So there is clearly a range of controlled movement speeds that are safe and productive for muscle development.

▶ **Recommendation:** You should perform strength training exercises at controlled movement speeds with minimum momentum. A good guideline is six seconds for each repetition (a two-second lifting phase and a four-second lowering phase).

You can exert more muscle force lowering the weightload than lifting the weightload. Therefore, to challenge your muscles during the lowering part of the exercise we recommend slowing down your movement speed. For example, a popular and proven training protocol is two seconds for the harder lifting phase and four seconds for the easier lowering phase of each repetition.

Although your training speed is largely a matter of personal preference, it is important to keep all exercise repetitions under control. One means for assessing your movement control is the stop test. When muscular force is moving the resistance, it is possible to stop the weightload at any point in the exercise range. If you can, you are using the right speed. When momentum is moving the resistance, it is not possible to stop the weightload at a particular point. Try this test during your exercises to see if you are working at a controlled speed.

Although faster movement speeds may be acceptable, repetitions requiring four seconds or longer have been shown to be safe and effective for strength development. We, therefore, encourage you to do strength training in a careful manner, paying close attention to control when lifting and lowering the weightload.

Movement Range

We recommend exercising through the *full range of joint movement* for two reasons. First, research indicates that full-range strength training enhances joint flexibility. Second, studies show that full-range exercise movements are necessary to develop full-range muscle strength.

Full range of joint movement—Exercising the muscle from the fully stretched position to the completely contracted position.

The importance of full-range muscle strength is underscored by extensive research with low back patients at the University of Florida Medical School. The researchers discovered that people with weak low back muscles were more likely to experience low back pain than people with strong low back muscles. They also determined that exercising the low back muscles through their full movement range was necessary for developing strength in all positions. This was an important finding because about 80 percent of the patients who increased their full-range back strength experienced less low back discomfort.

Although some people believe that strength training reduces joint flexibility, research with golfers over age 50 showed that eight weeks of full-range strength-training exercises did not decrease their movement range. And they significantly improved their club head speeds and driving power as a result of the strength-training program.

So what exactly is full-range strength-training exercise? Full-range strength-training exercise means training from the position of full muscle stretch to the position of full muscle contraction. Note that when the target muscle group (e.g., biceps) is fully contracted, the opposing muscle group (e.g., triceps) is fully stretched, and vice versa.

▶**Recommendation:** Whenever possible, perform strength-training exercises through your full range of joint movement.

Of course, you should not exceed normal joint limits or experience pain in any portion of the exercise movement. Eliminate or abbreviate exercises that cause joint discomfort, training only in the pain-free movement range.

Exercise Breathing

Regardless of the exercise effort, you should never hold your breath when performing strength-training exercises. Breath-holding may cause excessive internal pressure that restricts blood flow, resulting in lightheadedness and high blood pressure responses. Prevent these undesirable responses by breathing continuously during every exercise set.

▶**Recommendation:** Do *not* hold your breath during repetitions. Exhale when you lift the weightload and inhale when you lower the weightload.

Breathing out when you lift the weightload and breathing in when you lower the weightload maintains a more desirable internal air pressure. Because continuous breathing is a critical component of safe strength-training exercise, be sure to practice proper breathing on every repetition.

Program Factors

Program factors include

- activity order and
- warm-ups and cool-downs.

Activity Order

Strength-training exercise is best for improving muscular fitness, and aerobic exercise is best for improving cardiovascular fitness. But if you do both activities during the same training session, is it better to begin with strength-training exercise or endurance exercise?

In a study by one of the authors, 43 adults performed identical programs of strength-training exercises (10 machines) and endurance exercise (20 minutes of cycling, walking, or stepping), three days a week, for eight weeks. Half of the subjects always did the strength-training exercise first, and half of the subjects always did the endurance exercise first. As presented in table 6.4, both training groups experienced essentially equal strength increases after two months of exercise. Therefore, the order that you do strength-training exercise and endurance exercise is largely a matter of personal preference.

Table 6.4

STRENGTH GAIN AND WORKOUT ORDER

Training protocol (8 weeks)	Mean weight increase (11 Nautilus machines in pounds)
Strength exercise first	+22
Endurance exercise first	+23

▶ **Recommendation:** Perform strength-training exercise and endurance exercise in the order you prefer.

Of course if your primary goal is better strength fitness, it makes sense to perform strength training first. If your main objective is better cardiovascular fitness, it is logical to perform aerobic exercise first. Whichever activity you choose, however, be sure to begin each training session with a few minutes of warm-up exercise and conclude each training session with a few minutes of cool-down exercise. These transition phases between rest and vigorous physical activity provide important physiological and psychological benefits.

Warm-Ups and Cool-Downs

Strength training is high-effort exercise that places relatively heavy demands on your musculoskeletal system. Therefore,

For Lower Strength Levels

You may want to limit your workout to strength training only until your physical fitness improves. Don't add endurance exercises until you can complete your strength-training exercises without difficulty and undue fatigue.

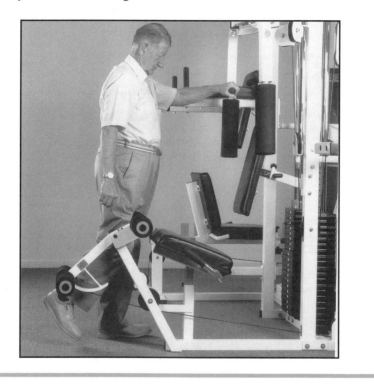

you should not jump right into a strength workout nor should you abruptly end a strength workout.

▶ **Recommendation:** You should begin and end your workouts with a few minutes of light activity to transition your muscles gradually from the resting state to the working state and vice versa.

Warm-ups and cool-downs should involve large muscle activity such as cycling, walking, or stepping. They may also include a few body-weight exercises such as knee bends, side bends, or trunk curls.

After strenuous activity blood tends to accumulate in the lower legs, which can cause undesirable changes in blood pressure and stress your cardiovascular system. Cool-downs facilitate blood flow to your heart and the smooth return to resting circulation. Recommended cool-down activities include easy cycling and walking, followed by gentle stretching exercises. It is usually sufficient to warm up and cool down 5 to 10 minutes.

SUMMARY OF STRENGTH-TRAINING PRINCIPLES AND PRACTICES

We recommend that you adhere to the following guidelines for safe and successful strength-training exercise.

TRAINING PRINCIPLES

Exercise Selection and Order

Train all of your major muscle groups to develop balanced strength throughout your muscular system. You should typically exercise your larger muscles first, and try to train your opposing muscle groups together.

Training Frequency

You should strength train two or three nonconsecutive days each week.

Exercise Sets

Begin your strength-training program with one set of each exercise. As you become more advanced, you may add a second or third set of exercise if you so desire.

Exercise Resistance

For most training purposes, you should use a weightload you can lift for 8 to 12 repetitions.

Exercise Repetitions

You should typically perform 8 to 12 repetitions in each exercise set, but occasionally perform more repetitions with lower resistance and fewer repetitions with higher resistance for variety.

Training Progression

Generally, you should raise your weightloads about 2.5 pounds whenever you complete 12 repetitions with proper form on two successive workouts.   *cont'd*

Training Effort

You may increase your training effort by doing more sets of a given exercise or by doing more exercises for a given muscle group.

TECHNIQUE FACTORS

Movement Speed

You should perform all strength-training exercises at moderate to slow speeds, always under control. A good guideline is to use six seconds for each repetition.

Movement Range

Whenever possible, perform strength exercise through your full range of joint movement, from a position of full muscle stretch to a position of complete muscle contraction.

Exercise Breathing

Do your best to breathe continuously during each repetition, exhaling when you lift the weightload and inhaling when you lower the weightload.

PROGRAM FACTORS

Activity Order

Perform strength training exercise and endurance exercise in the order you prefer.

Warm-Ups and Cool-Downs

You should precede strength training with 5 to 10 minutes of warm-up activity to gradually transition from rest to vigorous exercise. Likewise, you should conclude your strength workout with 5 to 10 minutes of cool-down activity to gradually transition from vigorous exercise to rest.

"Getting and keeping fit was more crucial to me after a severe leg and foot injury in 1986. After several years of chronic foot pain and a lingering depressed mood, I joined the YMCA and began . . . strength training three times a week. Since beginning that commitment in June of 1994, I am lighter in spirit [and] 23 pounds lighter in body weight, with much less pain. [I'm] dedicated to this routine for life."

—Beverly Moore, age 57

chapter 7

Working Out

By now you recognize that strength-training workouts are the building blocks that lead to better muscular fitness. Of course, the pathway you follow in your strength-training workouts should be systematic and geared toward progressive improvement. With this in mind, we have designed this chapter to provide you with sample strength-training workouts, whether you're a man or woman in your 50s, 60s, or 70s. We have based these workouts on the exercises featured in chapter 5 and the guidelines presented in chapter 6. You can tailor each to your personal level of strength fitness as determined in chapter 2. Your training program will begin with five basic exercises, and you will add new exercises during a 10-week period. And since we have included exercises for both machine and free-weight equipment, you may choose a workout program that suits your needs. If you have strength trained previously, you may be able to safely progress more quickly, but keep reasonably close to the recommended exercise protocol guidelines provided.

Suggested Workouts for Men and Women: Weeks 1 and 2

Your strength-training introductory sessions feature five standard exercises that involve most of your major muscle groups. If you choose a machine training program the exercises are the

- leg press for the front- and back-of-thigh muscles,
- chest press for the upper body pushing muscles,
- compound row for the upper body pulling muscles,
- abdominal curl for the midsection muscles, and
- back extension for the low back muscles.

If you prefer a free-weight training program, the exercises are the

- dumbbell squat for the front- and back-of-thigh muscles,
- dumbbell bench press for the upper body pushing muscles,
- dumbbell one-arm row for the upper body pulling muscles,
- dumbbell seated press for the shoulder muscles, and
- trunk curl for the midsection muscles.

We have based our suggestions for starting weightloads on our research involving Nautilus machines, and on our experience gained from our training and training others on free-weights. Please check your strength score for appropriate adjustments in the recommended exercise weightloads (see chapter 2). If your strength score was low, subtract 5 pounds from the suggested starting weightload. If your strength score was below average, subtract 2.5 pounds from the suggested starting weightload. If your strength score was above average, add 2.5 pounds to the suggested starting weightload, and if your strength score was high, add 5 pounds to the suggested starting weightload. Finally, for each exercise, be sure to review chapter 5 for proper technique.

Table 7.1 presents machine training information for men and women during weeks 1 and 2 of this strength program. Find the appropriate age category and make adjustments to the weightloads for each exercise based on your strength score (see chapter 2). Use Training Log 1 in appendix A to record your exercise weightloads and the number of repetitions you complete. For ease in writing in your entries, you may wish to photocopy and enlarge the training log. When you complete 12 repetitions with good form during two consecutive workouts, increase the exercise weightload by 2.5 pounds. Refer to figure 7.1, Sample Training Log, for assistance in filling out the log—

For Lower Strength Levels

Remember, if your test results indicate you have very low muscle strength, reduce the recommended starting resistance by 10 pounds or more. Also, rest at least three minutes between each exercise.

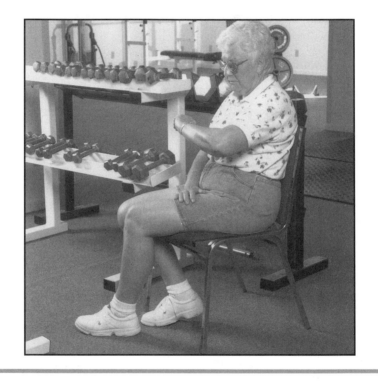

it shows where to record training dates, weightloads, reps completed, and comments about your workouts.

Table 7.2 provides free-weight training information for men and women during weeks 1 and 2 of this strength program. Find the appropriate age category and make adjustments to the weightloads for each exercise based on your strength score (see chapter 2). Record your exercise weightloads and the number of repetitions you complete on Training Log 2 in appendix A. When you complete 12 repetitions with good form during two consecutive workouts, increase the exercise weightload by 2.5 pounds.

Table 7.1

STRENGTH-TRAINING PROGRAM FOR WEEKS 1 AND 2

MACHINE TRAINING—MEN

New exercises	Muscle groups	STARTING WEIGHTLOAD FOR DIFFERENT AGE GROUPS*		
		50-59	60-69	70-79
Leg press	Front-of-thigh Back-of-thigh	110.0 lbs.	100.0 lbs.	90.0 lbs.
Chest press	Chest Shoulders Back-of-arm	50.0 lbs.	45.0 lbs.	40.0 lbs.
Compound row	Upper back Shoulders Front-of-arm	70.0 lbs.	62.5 lbs.	55.0 lbs.
Abdominal curl	Midsection	55.0 lbs.	50.0 lbs.	45.0 lbs.
Back extension	Lower back	55.0 lbs.	50.0 lbs.	45.0 lbs.

MACHINE TRAINING—WOMEN

New exercises	Muscle groups	STARTING WEIGHTLOAD FOR DIFFERENT AGE GROUPS*		
		50-59	60-69	70-79
Leg press	Front-of-thigh Back-of-thigh	75.0 lbs.	67.5 lbs.	60.0 lbs.
Chest press	Chest Shoulders Back-of-arm	32.5 lbs.	30.0 lbs.	27.5 lbs.
Compound row	Upper back Shoulders Front-of-arm	47.5 lbs.	42.5 lbs.	37.5 lbs.
Abdominal curl	Midsection	37.5 lbs.	35.0 lbs.	32.5 lbs.
Back extension	Lower back	37.5 lbs.	35.0 lbs.	32.5 lbs.

*Add or subtract the appropriate amount of resistance based on your chapter 2 strength score.

Low: -5.0 lbs.   Below avg: -2.5 lbs.   Above avg: +2.5 lbs.   High: +5.0 lbs.

Name _____

Training Log 1
Machine Exercises—Weeks 1 and 2

Order	Exercise	Reps/Sets	Set	Week #1 Day 1 1	2	3	Day 2 1	2	3	Day 3 1	2	3	Week #2 Day 1 1	2	3	Day 2 1	2	3	Day 3 1	2	3
1	Leg press	8-12 / 1	Wt.	100			100			100			102.5			102.5			105		
			Reps.	10			12			13			12			13			12		
2	Chest press	8-12 / 1	Wt.	47.5			47.5			50			50			50			52.5		
			Reps.	12			12			10			12			13			12		
3	Compound row	8-12 / 1	Wt.	62.5			62.5			62.5			62.5			65			65		
			Reps.	9			11			12			12			10			12		
4	Abdominal curl	8-12 / 1	Wt.	50			50			50			52.5			52.5			52.5		
			Reps.	11			12			12			11			12			13		
5	Back extension	8-12 / 1	Wt.	52.5			52.5			55			55			55			57.5		
			Reps.	13			14			11			12			12			11		
6			Wt.																		
			Reps.																		
7			Wt.																		
			Reps.																		
8			Wt.																		
			Reps.																		
9			Wt.																		
			Reps.																		
10			Wt.																		
			Reps.																		
11			Wt.																		
			Reps.																		
12			Wt.																		
			Reps.																		

Body weight
Date
Comments

Figure 7.1 Sample training log for basic programs.

Table 7.2

STRENGTH-TRAINING PROGRAM FOR WEEKS 1 AND 2

FREE-WEIGHT TRAINING—MEN

New exercises	Muscle groups	STARTING WEIGHTLOAD FOR DIFFERENT AGE GROUPS*		
		50-59	**60-69**	**70-79**
Dumbbell squat	Front-of-thigh Back-of-thigh	25.0 lbs.	20.0 lbs.	15.0 lbs.
Dumbbell bench press	Chest Shoulders Back-of-arm	25.0 lbs.	20.0 lbs.	15.0 lbs.
Dumbbell one-arm row	Upper back Shoulders Front-of-arm	25.0 lbs.	20.0 lbs.	15.0 lbs.
Dumbbell press	Shoulders	20.0 lbs.	15.0 lbs.	10.0 lbs.
Trunk curl	Midsection	20 reps	15 reps	10 reps

FREE-WEIGHT TRAINING—WOMEN

New exercises	Muscle groups	STARTING WEIGHTLOAD FOR DIFFERENT AGE GROUPS*		
		50-59	**60-69**	**70-79**
Dumbbell squat	Front-of-thigh Back-of-thigh	15.0 lbs.	12.5 lbs.	10.0 lbs.
Dumbbell bench press	Chest Shoulders Back-of-arm	12.5 lbs.	10.0 lbs.	7.5 lbs.
Dumbbell one-arm row	Upper back Shoulders Front-of-arm	12.5 lbs.	10.0 lbs.	7.5 lbs.
Dumbbell press	Shoulders	12.5 lbs.	10.0 lbs.	7.5 lbs.
Trunk curl	Midsection	15 reps	10 reps	5 reps

*Add or subtract the appropriate amount of resistance based on your chapter 2 strength score.

Low: -5.0 lbs.   Below avg: -2.5 lbs.   Above avg: +2.5 lbs.   High: +5.0 lbs.

You may wish to photocopy the training logs in this book so that you can use them over and over. In addition, you do not have to use every column or exercise in the training logs in appendix A. Tailor your use of the training logs as you tailor your workouts to meet your needs.

Suggested Workouts for Men and Women: Weeks 3 and 4

Congratulations on completing two weeks of strength training! You are strengthening most of your major muscle groups and the weightloads are beginning to feel lighter. Because many adults are concerned about hip function, we suggest that you add two exercises if the machines you need for them are available. These are the hip adduction machine for your inner thigh muscles, and the hip abduction machine for your outer thigh muscles. Do these exercises after the leg press, and continue performing the chest press, compound row, abdominal curl, and back extension in this order, concentrating on good form.

If you are training with free weights, the squat exercise is an excellent hip strengthener, so you need not add other lower body exercises at this time. Instead, complement your workout with dumbbell curls for the front-of-arm muscles (biceps) and dumbbell overhead triceps extensions for the back-of-arm muscles (triceps). Keep doing your other free-weight exercises, inserting the new arm exercises right before your trunk curls.

Table 7.3 gives machine training information for men and women during weeks 3 and 4 of this strength program. Find the appropriate age category and make adjustments to the weightloads for each exercise based on your strength score (see chapter 2). Record your exercise weightloads and the number of repetitions you complete on Training Log 3 in appendix A. When you complete 12 repetitions with good form during two consecutive workouts, increase the exercise weightload by 2.5 pounds.

Table 7.4 presents free-weight training information for men and women during weeks 3 and 4 of this strength program. Find the appropriate age category and make adjustments to

Table 7.3

STRENGTH-TRAINING PROGRAM FOR WEEKS 3 AND 4

MACHINE TRAINING—MEN

New exercises	Muscle groups	STARTING WEIGHTLOAD FOR DIFFERENT AGE GROUPS*		
		50-59	60-69	70-79
Hip adduction	Inner thigh	65.0 lbs.	60.0 lbs.	55.0 lbs.
Hip abduction	Outer thigh	55.0 lbs.	50.0 lbs.	45.0 lbs.

MACHINE TRAINING—WOMEN

New exercises	Muscle groups	STARTING WEIGHTLOAD FOR DIFFERENT AGE GROUPS*		
		50-59	60-69	70-79
Hip adduction	Inner thigh	47.5 lbs.	45.0 lbs.	42.5 lbs.
Hip abduction	Outer thigh	37.5 lbs.	35.0 lbs.	32.5 lbs.

*Add or subtract the appropriate amount of resistance based on your chapter 2 strength score.

Low: -5.0 lbs.   Below avg: -2.5 lbs.   Above avg: +2.5 lbs.   High: +5.0 lbs.

the weightloads for each exercise based on your strength score (see chapter 2). Record your exercise weightloads and the number of repetitions you complete on Training Log 4 in appendix A. When you complete 12 repetitions with good form during two consecutive workouts, increase the exercise weightload by 2.5 pounds.

Suggested Workouts for Men and Women: Weeks 5 and 6

Your machine training involves three exercises for your legs, two exercises for your trunk, and two exercises for your upper

Table 7.4

STRENGTH-TRAINING PROGRAM FOR WEEKS 3 AND 4

FREE-WEIGHT TRAINING—MEN

New exercises	Muscle groups	STARTING WEIGHTLOAD FOR DIFFERENT AGE GROUPS*		
		50-59	**60-69**	**70-79**
Dumbbell curl	Front-of-arm	15.0 lbs.	12.5 lbs.	10.0 lbs.
Dumbbell overhead triceps extension	Back-of arm	20.0 lbs.	17.5 lbs.	15.0 lbs.

FREE-WEIGHT TRAINING—WOMEN

New exercises	Muscle groups	STARTING WEIGHTLOAD FOR DIFFERENT AGE GROUPS*		
		50-59	**60-69**	**70-79**
Dumbbell curl	Front-of-arm	10.0 lbs.	7.5 lbs.	5.0 lbs.
Dumbbell overhead triceps extension	Back-of arm	12.5 lbs.	10.0 lbs.	7.5 lbs.

*Add or subtract the appropriate amount of resistance based on your chapter 2 strength score.

Low: -5.0 lbs.   Below avg: -2.5 lbs.   Above avg: +2.5 lbs.   High: +5.0 lbs.

body. Although your arms are involved in both the chest press and compound row exercises, you may train them more directly with triceps extensions and biceps curls. The triceps extension machine targets your back-of-arm muscles (triceps), and the biceps curl machine targets your front-of-arm muscles (biceps). During this training period add these two exercises between the compound row and abdominal curl. In all exercises, be sure to increase the weightload by 2.5 pounds whenever you complete 12 repetitions with good form during two consecutive workouts.

If you are training with free weights, add the dumbbell shrug for your shoulders and the dumbbell heel raise for the back of your lower leg (calf). Do these new exercises after all the other exercises, which you should continue to perform in the same order. Whenever you complete 12 repetitions with good form during two consecutive workouts, increase the weightload by 2.5 pounds.

Table 7.5 provides machine training information for men and women during weeks 5 and 6 of this strength program. Find the appropriate age category and make adjustments to the weightloads for each exercise based on your strength score (chapter 2). Record your exercise weightloads and the number of repetitions you complete on Training Log 5 in appendix A.

Table 7.6 offers free-weight training information for men and women during weeks 5 and 6 of this strength program.

Table 7.5

STRENGTH-TRAINING PROGRAM FOR WEEKS 5 AND 6

MACHINE TRAINING—MEN

New exercises	Muscle groups	STARTING WEIGHTLOAD FOR DIFFERENT AGE GROUPS*		
		50-59	**60-69**	**70-79**
Triceps extension	Back-of-arm	45.0 lbs.	40.0 lbs.	35.0 lbs.
Biceps curl	Front-of-arm	45.0 lbs.	40.0 lbs.	35.0 lbs.

MACHINE TRAINING—WOMEN

New exercises	Muscle groups	STARTING WEIGHTLOAD FOR DIFFERENT AGE GROUPS*		
		50-59	**60-69**	**70-79**
Triceps extension	Back-of-arm	25.0 lbs.	22.5 lbs.	20.0 lbs.
Biceps curl	Front-of-arm	25.0 lbs.	22.5 lbs.	20.0 lbs.

*Add or subtract the appropriate amount of resistance based on your chapter 2 strength score.
Low: -5.0 lbs.   Below avg: -2.5 lbs.   Above avg: +2.5 lbs.   High: +5.0 lbs.

Table 7.6

STRENGTH-TRAINING PROGRAM FOR WEEKS 5 AND 6

FREE-WEIGHT TRAINING—MEN

New exercises	Muscle groups	STARTING WEIGHTLOAD FOR DIFFERENT AGE GROUPS*		
		50-59	60-69	70-79
Dumbbell shrug	Shoulders	25.0 lbs.	20.0 lbs.	15.0 lbs.
Dumbbell heel raise	Calf	25.0 lbs.	20.0 lbs.	15.0 lbs.

FREE-WEIGHT TRAINING—WOMEN

New exercises	Muscle groups	STARTING WEIGHTLOAD FOR DIFFERENT AGE GROUPS*		
		50-59	60-69	70-79
Dumbbell shrug	Shoulders	15.0 lbs.	12.5 lbs.	10.0 lbs.
Dumbbell heel raise	Calf	15.0 lbs.	12.5 lbs.	10.0 lbs.

*Add or subtract the appropriate amount of resistance based on your chapter 2 strength score.
Low: -5.0 lbs.   Below avg: -2.5 lbs.   Above avg: +2.5 lbs.   High: +5.0 lbs.

Find the appropriate age category and make adjustments to the weightloads for each exercise based on your strength score (chapter 2). Record your exercise weightloads and the number of repetitions you complete on Training Log 6 in appendix A.

Suggested Workouts for Men and Women: Weeks 7 and 8

After six weeks of regular strength training you should notice some major improvements in your body composition, namely, more muscle and less fat. You should also feel stronger than you have for years. If you are using machines, replace the chest press and compound row with three exercises that better target your chest, upper back, and shoulder muscles. The new machine exercises are the chest crossover, super-pullover, and lateral raise. As usual, increase your exercise weightloads by 2.5 pounds whenever you complete 12 repetitions with good form during two consecutive workouts.

If you are using free weights, complement the dumbbell bench press exercise for chest development by adding the dumbbell chest fly exercise. This exercise better isolates your chest muscles. It should be performed after the dumbbell bench press exercise.

Table 7.7 presents machine training information for men and women during weeks 7 and 8 of this strength program. Find the appropriate age category and make adjustments to the weightloads for each exercise based on your strength score (chapter 2). Record your exercise weightloads and the number of repetitions you complete on Training Log 7 in appendix A.

Table 7.8 offers free-weight training information for men and women during weeks 7 and 8 of this strength program. Find the appropriate age category and make adjustments to the weightloads for each exercise based on your strength score (see chapter 2). Record your exercise weightloads and the number of repetitions you complete on Training Log 8 in appendix A.

Table 7.7

STRENGTH-TRAINING PROGRAM FOR WEEKS 7 AND 8

MACHINE TRAINING—MEN

New exercises	Muscle groups	STARTING WEIGHTLOAD FOR DIFFERENT AGE GROUPS*		
		50-59	60-69	70-79
Chest crossover	Chest	52.5 lbs.	50.0 lbs.	47.5 lbs.
Super-pullover	Upper back	57.5 lbs.	55.0 lbs.	52.5 lbs.
Lateral raise	Shoulders	47.5 lbs.	45.0 lbs.	42.5 lbs.

MACHINE TRAINING—WOMEN

New exercises	Muscle groups	STARTING WEIGHTLOAD FOR DIFFERENT AGE GROUPS*		
		50-59	**60-69**	**70-79**
Chest crossover	Chest	30.0 lbs.	27.5 lbs.	25.0 lbs.
Super-pullover	Upper back	32.5 lbs.	30.0 lbs.	27.5 lbs.
Lateral raise	Shoulders	27.5 lbs.	25.0 lbs.	22.5 lbs.

*Add or subtract the appropriate amount of resistance based on your chapter 2 strength score.

Low: -5.0 lbs.　Below avg: -2.5 lbs.　Above avg: +2.5 lbs.　High: +5.0 lbs.

Table 7.8

STRENGTH-TRAINING PROGRAM FOR WEEKS 7 AND 8

FREE-WEIGHT TRAINING—MEN

New exercises	Muscle groups	STARTING WEIGHTLOAD FOR DIFFERENT AGE GROUPS*		
		50-59	**60-69**	**70-79**
Dumbbell chest fly	Chest	15.0 lbs.	12.5 lbs.	10.0 lbs.

FREE-WEIGHT TRAINING—WOMEN

New exercises	Muscle groups	STARTING WEIGHTLOAD FOR DIFFERENT AGE GROUPS*		
		50-59	**60-69**	**70-79**
Dumbbell chest fly	Chest	10.0 lbs.	7.5 lbs.	5.0 lbs.

*Add or subtract the appropriate amount of resistance based on your chapter 2 strength score.

Low: -5.0 lbs.　Below avg: -2.5 lbs.　Above avg: +2.5 lbs.　High: +5.0 lbs.

Suggested Workouts for Men and Women: Weeks 9 and 10

Just as you changed the upper body machine exercises to better target your chest, upper back, and shoulder muscles, you can now do the same to better isolate your leg muscles. Replace the leg press with the leg extension and leg curl exercises. The leg extension addresses the front-of-thigh muscles, and the leg curl addresses the back-of-thigh muscles. You should continue to increase your exercise weightloads by 2.5 pounds whenever you complete 12 repetitions with good form during two consecutive workouts.

If you are using free weights you may have access to a pulley apparatus on which you can do lat pull-downs for your upper back muscles and triceps press-downs for your back-of-arm muscles. We recommend that you substitute these exercises for the dumbbell one-arm row and the dumbbell overhead triceps extension. The pulley exercises provide excellent training for these muscle groups and add variety to your workout program. If you do not have access to this equipment, continue doing the dumbbell one-arm row and dumbbell overhead triceps extension exercises.

Table 7.9 presents machine training information for men and women during weeks 9 and 10 of this strength program. Find the appropriate age category and make adjustments to the weightloads for each exercise based on your strength score (see chapter 2). Record your exercise weightloads and the number of repetitions you complete on Training Log 9 in appendix A.

Table 7.10 provides free-weight training information for men and women during weeks 9 and 10 of this strength program. Find the appropriate age category and make adjustments to the weightloads for each exercise based on your strength score (see chapter 2). Record your exercise weightloads and the number of repetitions you complete on Training Log 10 in appendix A. When you complete 12 repetitions with good form during two consecutive workouts, increase the exercise weightload by 2.5 pounds.

Table 7.9

STRENGTH-TRAINING PROGRAM FOR WEEKS 9 AND 10

MACHINE TRAINING—MEN

New exercises	Muscle groups	STARTING WEIGHTLOAD FOR DIFFERENT AGE GROUPS*		
		50-59	60-69	70-79
Leg extension	Front-of-thigh	55.0 lbs.	50.0 lbs.	45.0 lbs.
Leg curl	Back-of-thigh	55.0 lbs.	50.0 lbs.	45.0 lbs.

MACHINE TRAINING—WOMEN

New exercises	Muscle groups	STARTING WEIGHTLOAD FOR DIFFERENT AGE GROUPS*		
		50-59	60-69	70-79
Leg extension	Front-of-thigh	35.0 lbs.	30.0 lbs.	25.0 lbs.
Leg curl	Back-of-thigh	35.0 lbs.	30.0 lbs.	25.0 lbs.

*Add or subtract the appropriate amount of resistance based on your chapter 2 strength score.

Low: -5.0 lbs.   Below avg: -2.5 lbs.   Above avg: +2.5 lbs.   High: +5.0 lbs.

Summary

Congratulations! You have now completed 10 weeks of regular strength-training exercises. You are working all your major muscle groups productively and progressively, and the results should be obvious. At this point you have many options for continuing or changing your strength-training program. For example, you may alternate different exercises for your target muscles, thereby creating training variety. In fact, you may combine machine and free-weight training exercises if you so desire.

Table 7.10
STRENGTH-TRAINING PROGRAM FOR WEEKS 9 AND 10

FREE-WEIGHT TRAINING—MEN

New exercises	Muscle groups	STARTING WEIGHTLOAD FOR DIFFERENT AGE GROUPS*		
		50-59	60-69	70-79
Lat pull-down	Upper back Front-of-arm	60.0 lbs.	50.0 lbs.	40.0 lbs.
Triceps press-down	Back-of-arm	35.0 lbs.	30.0 lbs.	25.0 lbs.

FREE-WEIGHT TRAINING—WOMEN

New exercises	Muscle groups	STARTING WEIGHTLOAD FOR DIFFERENT AGE GROUPS*		
		50-59	60-69	70-79
Lateral pull-down	Upper back Front-of-arm	40.0 lbs.	35.0 lbs.	30.0 lbs.
Triceps press-down	Back-of-arm	25.0 lbs.	20.0 lbs.	15.0 lbs.

*Add or subtract the appropriate amount of resistance based on your chapter 2 strength score.
Low: -5.0 lbs.   Below avg: -2.5 lbs.   Above avg: +2.5 lbs.   High: +5.0 lbs.

If you have the time and desire to expand your strength-training workouts, you may perform more sets of each exercise or additional exercises for each major muscle group. You may also use different training protocols to emphasize larger muscle size, greater muscle strength, or more muscle endurance. In chapter 8, we will show you how to design an advanced strength-training program that works for you.

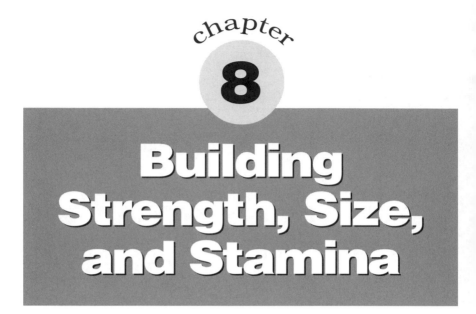

chapter

8

Building Strength, Size, and Stamina

The 10-week training program we described in chapter 7 is a basic one that gradually introduces you to some important exercises and the loads, repetitions, and sets to use with them. The systematic integration of these elements gives you the opportunity to master the techniques involved in the exercises and to adapt physiologically to the training. Assuming that you have been following and are nearing the end of the 10-week program, you may be wondering what you should do next. Well, that's up to you. You may choose to continue following your current workout because you are happy with the improvements you've made in strength and how your body is looking. If so, continue to train as you have been, adding to your weightloads when you are able to perform more than 12 reps of an exercise on two consecutive workout occasions.

Taking the Challenge

You may, however, decide to try more challenging workouts. If so, this can be an exciting time! Your body is capable of handling heavier loads, and your muscular endurance has improved to a point at which you can endure longer and more intense workouts. In fact, you are not only capable of adding weight to the exercises in your program but also of increasing the number of sets and exercises you perform. Of course, the advantage of undertaking more strenuous workouts is that they will produce even greater gains than those you've already experienced. Add to this the opportunity to select from three programs (muscle size, muscle strength, or muscle endurance) that enable you to accomplish specific goals, and you have some exciting options to consider. Just be sensible in your approach to more and harder strength-training exercise by progressing gradually, maintaining proper form, and always working within your ability level.

Should you decide to take the challenge, you will need to establish a primary goal for training. Will your goal be to

- increase muscle size,
- increase muscle strength, or
- increase muscle endurance?

Once you choose a program, refer to the appropriate section and follow the workouts presented. As in chapter 7, you will have a choice between free-weight and machine workouts. If you decide to combine free-weight and machine exercises in your workouts, refer to chapter 6 for guidance and adapt the training logs in appendix B to accommodate the changes you make. Remember, feel free to photocopy the training logs in this book so that you can use them over and over.

About the Advanced Programs in This Chapter

Because the program options we'll present next build on the 10-week program of exercises that you are now following, you can use the strength and endurance you have acquired to handle more demanding workouts. To reduce the chances of injury caused by doing too much too soon, each program presented in this chapter begins with a four-week transition period. Following the transition period are two additional four-week programs (sometimes referred to as "training cycles"), each of which increases in training intensity.

Not surprisingly, as the workouts in these programs become more demanding, the time required to complete them also increases. So to assist you with scheduling your training sessions, we have listed the approximate amount of time you'll need to set aside for completing them at the bottom of each program. Note that we have made an effort to keep the workouts short but still effective. If your time is especially limited, however, you may elect to use the transition period (weeks 11 through 14) as your standard training cycle because it takes less time than those in weeks 15 through 22. If so, remember to increase training loads by 2.5 pounds whenever you are able to perform more than the designated number of reps in two consecutive workout sessions.

The following directions and explanations will help you understand how to adapt your current training approach to the more advanced training cycles shown in Training Logs 11 through 16. Before deciding which program you will follow, consider the equipment requirements of the training exercises. Also note that the free-weight barbell squat, heel raise, and bench press exercises require spotters for safe and effective performance.

Whichever program you choose, be sure to do the following:

- Record the weightloads you plan to use and the number of reps you intend to do ("goal reps") in the training logs in appendix B as you did in appendix A (see also figure 8.1 at the end of this chapter).

- Perform exercises in the order in which they are listed.

- Modify starting loads as described.

- Try to perform the number of repetitions indicated, expecting that the number of reps you will be able to complete in the second and third sets will be fewer than those in the first set.

- When doing more than one set of an exercise, increase the weightload by 2.5 lbs. whenever you complete the specified number of repetitions in the first set on two successive workouts.

1. If you cannot perform the correct number of repetitions, adjust loads using the load adjustment guidelines provided in table 8.1.

2. If using the free-weight programs, decide if you will opt to use a barbell in some of the exercises (listed with an asterisk in the training logs). If you decide to use a barbell, you will need to increase the loads you are using in your dumbbell exercises, but by how much? Simply double the dumbbell weight (weight of one dumbbell) you are using in the same exercise, and then adjust according to table 8.1.

3. If you decide to add additional exercises or perform more sets later, and especially if you decide to do both, consider going to a four-day-a-week program. A four-day-a-week program (called a "split program") splits up your exercises so that you do some two days a week (e.g., Monday and Thursday) and others on two other days (e.g., Tuesday and Friday). If you are considering this approach, refer to the books *Essentials of Strength Training and Conditioning* by Baechle (1994), or *Weight Training: Steps to Success* by Baechle and Groves (1997) for more detailed explanations of split program training. The purpose of splitting exercise sessions into smaller segments is to reduce the workout time and to provide a longer recovery period for the muscles trained twice a week. This enables your body to better tolerate the harder training program and lessens the likelihood of overtraining.

• Record the results of each workout in the appropriate training log in appendix B.

Workouts That Emphasize Muscle Size

We have adapted your current program in the following ways:

• The number of repetitions you'll do for Training Logs 11 and 12 is 8 to 12 per exercise, which means you will need to

Table 8.1

LOAD ADJUSTMENT GUIDELINES FOR REPETITIONS COMPLETED

Reps	Below goal subtract	Above goal add
1	2.5 pounds	2.5 pounds
2	5 pounds	5 pounds
3	7.5 pounds	7.5 pounds
4	10 pounds	10 pounds
5	12.5 pounds	12.5 pounds
6	15 pounds	15 pounds

In the left hand column identify the number of reps that you performed below or above the "goal rep" number listed in your training log for a particular exercise. If you performed too few, subtract the number of pounds listed beneath the column titled "Below goal" from your current weightload. In the same manner add the poundage shown beneath the column heading "Above goal" if you performed too many reps.

increase weightloads (see tables 8.2, *a* and *b*). Add five pounds to the exercises in your current program. Increasing your weightload will reduce the number of repetitions you can complete, putting you in the lower end of the rep range of 8 to 12. Your 10 weeks of training leading up to the workouts in Training Logs 11 through 16 have prepared you well for these heavier weightloads. However, if you are not confident about increasing weightloads by 5 pounds all at once, you may want to add 2.5 pounds in week 11 and another 2.5 pounds in week 12.

• We have added an arm muscle exercise—the barbell curl in the free-weight program and the weight-assisted pull-up in the machine program. If you choose to use barbells, double the weight you are currently using in the dumbbell curl. In the weight-assisted pull-up machine exercise, try using 40 percent of your body weight if you're male, 60 percent if you're female. The weightload in this exercise is used to counterbalance your own weight, so adding weight makes it easier to perform. Again, use table 8.1 as needed to make load adjustments. We encourage you to add different exercises if you would like to emphasize a muscle area other than the arms.

• We have increased the number of sets in certain exercises to two for the first four weeks, then three in the last four weeks. In other exercises the number of sets increases to two during the second four-week cycle and remains at two in the third cycle (see tables 8.2, *a* and *b*).

• Rest periods are now one to two minutes instead of only one minute.

• Make it your goal to perform 30 reps in both sets of the trunk curl during weeks 11 through 14, 35 reps in weeks 15 through 18, and 40 reps in weeks 19 through 22.

• After week 22 your body will benefit from a week of less intense training. So at this point, perform only one set of 8 to 12 reps of each exercise. During the following week resume the workout you were following in Training Log 11 or 12 and table 8.2*a* or table 8.2*b*, picking up where you left off at the end of week 22 and making appropriate load adjustments. Thereafter, plan a less intense week of training during the eighth week of every training cycle.

Table 8.2a

MACHINE PROGRAM FOR MUSCLE SIZE DEVELOPMENT

Order	Exercise	WEEKS GOAL	Reps	11-14 Sets	15-18 Sets	19-22 Sets
1	Leg extension		8-12	2	3	3
2	Leg curl		8-12	2	3	3
3	Chest crossover		8-12	2	2	3
4	Chest press		8-12	2	3	3
5	Compound row		8-12	2	2	3
6	Lateral raise		8-12	1	2	2
7	Triceps extension		8-12	1	2	2
8	Biceps curl		8-12	2	3	3
9	Weight-assisted pull-up		8-12	1	2	2
10	Back extension		8-12	1	2	2
11	Abdominal curl		8-12	1	2	2
	Estimated time requirement (mins.)			*41*	*62*	*67*

Table 8.2b

FREE-WEIGHT PROGRAM FOR MUSCLE SIZE DEVELOPMENT

				11-14	15-18	19-22
		WEEKS				
Order	Exercise	GOAL	Reps	Sets	Sets	Sets
1	Dumbbell or barbell squat	8-12	1	2	2	
2	Dumbbell or barbell bench press	8-12	2	2	3	
3	Dumbbell chest fly	8-12	1	2	2	
4	Dumbbell one-arm row	8-12	2	2	2	
5	Dumbbell seated press	8-12	2	2	3	
6	Dumbbell lateral raise	8-12	1	2	2	
7	Barbell curl	8-12	2	2	2	
8	Dumbbell concentration curl	8-12	1	2	2	
9	Dumbbell overhead triceps extension	8-12	1	2	2	
10	Barbell shrug	8-12	1	2	2	
11	Abdominal curl	30	2	2	2	
	Estimated time requirement (mins.)			44	57	66

Workouts That Emphasize Strength Development

We have adapted your current program in the following ways:

• We have changed the number of repetitions in the workouts you'll do for Training Logs 11 through 22 to 5 to 8 in the exercises marked with an asterisk (see tables 8.3, *a* and *b*). To put yourself in the rep range of 5 to 8 for the four exercises with an asterisk, add 10 pounds to what you are currently using. If adding 10 pounds fails to put you in the rep range of 5 to 8, make appropriate weightload adjustments using figure 8.1 as a guide. For other exercises in the workout, you should perform 12 repetitions, again referring to figure 8.1. Once more, your muscles should be well-prepared for heavier weightloads that will provide a greater strength-building stimulus.

• We have increased the number of sets for the exercises in the rep range of 5 to 8 to two during the second four-week cycle, then to three during the last four-week cycle in those exercises with an asterisk. In the 12-rep exercises the number of sets increases to two during the *first* four-week cycle and remains at two throughout the second and third cycles (see tables 8.3, *a* and *b*).

• After week 22 your body will benefit from a week of less intense training. Perform only *one* set of each exercise and do the number of reps (5 to 8 or 12) listed for each exercise. During the following week, resume the workout you were following in Training Logs 13 or 14 and table 8.3*a* or table 8.3*b*, picking up where you left off at the end of week 22 and making appropriate weightload adjustments. Thereafter, plan a less intense week of training during the eighth week of every training cycle.

• Increase the length of your rest periods in between sets to three minutes. Longer rest periods allow more time for your muscles to recover more fully when using heavier loads, thus reducing the risk of overtraining and enabling your muscles to exert maximum effort during succeeding sets.

Table 8.3a

MACHINE PROGRAM FOR STRENGTH DEVELOPMENT

Order	Exercise	WEEKS GOAL	Reps	11-14 Sets	15-18 Sets	19-22 Sets
1	*Leg press		5-8	1	2	3
2	Heel raise		12	2	2	2
3	*Chest press		5-8	1	2	3
4	*Compound row		5-8	1	2	3
5	Lateral raise		12	2	2	2
6	Triceps extension		12	2	2	2
7	Back extension		8-12	2	3	3
8	Abdominal curl		12	2	2	2
	Estimated time requirement (mins.)			56	72	88

Table 8.3b

FREE-WEIGHT PROGRAM FOR STRENGTH DEVELOPMENT

Order	Exercise	WEEKS GOAL	Reps	11-14 Sets	15-18 Sets	19-22 Sets
1	Dumbbell or barbell squat	5-8		1	2	3
2	Dumbbell or barbell heel raise	12		2	2	2
3	Dumbbell or barbell bench press	5-8		1	2	3
4	Dumbbell one-arm row	5-8		1	2	3
5	Dumbbell seated press	5-8		1	2	3
6	Barbell curl	12		2	2	2
7	Dumbbell overhead triceps extension	12		2	2	2
8	Trunk curl	30		2	2	2
	Estimated time requirement (mins.)			*50*	*66*	*82*

Workouts That Emphasize Muscle Endurance

We have adapted your current program in the following ways:

• We have increased the number of repetitions you'll do for Training Logs 15 and 16 from 12 to 15 (see tables 8.4, *a* and *b*).

• Rather than reduce the loads you're lifting currently so you can perform more repetitions, progressively increase your reps to 15 at the same weight. Once you can do 16 or more repetitions in the first set on two consecutive occasions, increase the load by 2.5 pounds.

• We have increased the number of sets performed in certain exercises to two in the first four-week cycle, then to three during the last four-week cycle. In other exercises the number of sets increases to two during the second four-week cycle and remains at two in the third cycle (see tables 8.4, *a* and *b*).

• Rest periods of one minute remain the same.

• Make it your goal to perform 30 reps in both sets of the trunk curl during weeks 11 through 14, 35 reps in weeks 15 through 18, and 40 reps in weeks 19 through 22.

• After week 22 your body will benefit from a week of less intense training. Perform only *one* set of 15 reps in each exercise. During the following week, resume the workout you were following in Training Log 15 or 16 and table 8.4*a* or table 8.4*b*, picking up where you left off at the end of week 22 and making appropriate load adjustments. Thereafter, plan a less intense week of training during the eighth week of every training cycle.

If Your Goal Is Improved Body Composition

If reproportioning your body is your primary goal, it is likely that you believe you are carrying too much fat, not enough muscle or both. Consider one or all of these three actions to help you achieve a better body composition:

• Follow the muscle size program we described earlier in this chapter to increase muscle mass.

• Select foods more carefully for reduced fat and calorie intake (refer to chapter 9).

• Begin an aerobic (endurance) program to burn more calories. For additional guidance in this area refer to the texts *Fitness Weight Training* by Baechle and Earle (1995) and *Building Strength and Stamina* by Westcott (1996).

Recording Workout Information in the Training Logs

Once you have decided which program (muscle size, muscle strength, or muscle endurance) and which type of equipment you'll be using, the next step is to record your workout information in one of the six training logs located in appendix

Table 8.4a

MACHINE PROGRAM FOR MUSCLE ENDURANCE

		WEEKS		11-14	15-18	19-22
Order	Exercise	GOAL	Reps	Sets	Sets	Sets
1	Leg extension	15	2	2	3
2	Leg curl	15	2	2	3
3	Hip abduction	15	1	2	2
4	Hip adduction	15	1	2	2
5	Chest crossover	15	2	2	3
6	Super-pullover	15	2	2	3
7	Lateral raise	15	1	2	2
8	Triceps extension	15	1	2	2
9	Biceps curl	15	2	2	3
10	Rotary torso	15	1	2	2
	Estimated time requirement (mins.)			40	55	68

Table 8.4b

FREE-WEIGHT PROGRAM FOR MUSCLE ENDURANCE

		WEEKS		11-14	15-18	19-22
Order	Exercise	GOAL	Reps	Sets	Sets	Sets
1	Dumbbell or barbell squat	15	2	2	3
2	Dumbbell or barbell heel raise	15	1	2	2
3	Dumbbell or barbell bench press	15	2	2	3
4	Dumbbell chest fly	15	1	2	2
5	Dumbbell one-arm row	15	2	2	3
6	Dumbbell seated press	15	2	2	3
7	Barbell curl	15	2	2	3
8	Dumbbell overhead triceps extension	15	1	2	2
9	Barbell shrug	15	1	2	2
10	Trunk curl	30	2	2	2
	Estimated time requirement (mins.)			44	54	70

B. Simply identify the training log that has both the exercise program and the equipment that you'll be using (located at the top of the form). You can make six copies of this form if you intend to follow all three four-week training cycles; make more copies if you intend to repeat these workouts. Enlarging the logs as you copy them will make it easier for you to read and fill them out. Then using figure 8.1 as an example, simply transfer information regarding "goal reps," number of sets to perform, and weightloads. Figure 8.1 also shows where to record training dates, reps completed, and comments about your workouts.

"I have always considered fitness to be an essential part of my daily activities. This balanced approach to exercise has given me the energy reserves to cope with the daily . . . stresses of family life and my work for 22 years as a United States Air Force officer. More recently, in my new career as a personal trainer, I have renewed my emphasis on strength training, and as a result, I have been able to more effectively isolate muscle groups. By using the high-intensity training method, I've successfully achieved higher strength plateaus for specificity in sports activities, including qualifying for an international military triathlon and competing in the Scottish Highland Games athletic events throughout the United States and Hawaii."

—J.F. (Ian) Dargin, age 54
Major, USAF (Ret.)
Personal Trainer

Name Norman Bailer

Write in number of sets to perform here.

Write in "Goal reps" here

Write in weightload here.

Record number of reps completed here.

Write in the number of the training week.

Write in comments about your workouts, how you feel, and so on.

Order	Exercise	Reps / Sets	Set	Week # 11 Day 1 (1, 2, 3)	Week # 11 Day 2 (1, 2, 3)	Week # 11 Day 3 (1, 2, 3)	Week # 12 Day 1 (1, 2, 3)	Week # 12 Day 2 (1, 2, 3)	Week # 12 Day 3 (1, 2, 3)
1	Leg extension	8-12 / 2	Wt.	70, 70	70, 70	70, 70	70, 70	72.5, 72.5	72.5, 72.5
			Reps.	10, 9	10, 9	12, 11	13, 12	11, 8	11, 9
2	Leg curl	8-12 / 2	Wt.	60, 60	60, 60	60, 60	60, 60	60, 60	62.5, 62.5
			Reps.	10, 8	10, 9	10, 10	12, 11	13, 11	12, 11
3	Chest crossover	8-12 / 2	Wt.	80, 80	80, 80	80, 80	80, 80	80, 80	80, 80
			Reps.	10, 8	10, 9	10, 10	11, 11	12, 11	14, 12
4	Chest press	8-12 / 1	Wt.	62.5	62.5	62.5			
			Reps.	12	13	10	11		
5	Compound row	8-12 / 2	Wt.	65, 65	65, 65	65, 65	65, 65	67.5, 67.5	67.5, 67.5
			Reps.	10, 10	11, 11	12, 11	12, 12	10, 8	10, 9
6	Lateral raise	8-12 / 2	Wt.	60, 60	60, 60	60, 60	62.5, 62.5	62.5, 62.5	62.5, 62.5
			Reps.	11, 11	12, 11	13, 12	9, 8	10, 10	12, 11
7	Triceps extension	8-12 / 1	Wt.	60	60	60	60	62.5	62.5
			Reps.	8	10	10	13	13	14
8	Biceps curl	8-12 / 1	Wt.	65	65	65	65	65	65
			Reps.	10	10	11	12	14	14
9	Weight-assisted pull-ups	8-12 / 1	Wt.	50.0	50.0	50.0	50.0	50.0	50.0
			Reps.	9	10	11	11	12	14
10	Back extension	8-12 / 2	Wt.	57.5, 57.5	57.5, 57.5	57.5, 57.5	57.5, 57.5	57.5, 57.5	57.5, 57.5
			Reps.	9, 8	10, 9	10, 10	11, 10	12, 11	13, 12
11	Abdominal curl	8-12 / 1	Wt.	60	60	60	60	62.5	62.5
			Reps.	10	11	12	12	11	12
12			Wt.						
			Reps.						
	Body weight								
	Date								
	Comments								

Figure 8.1   Sample training log for advanced programs.

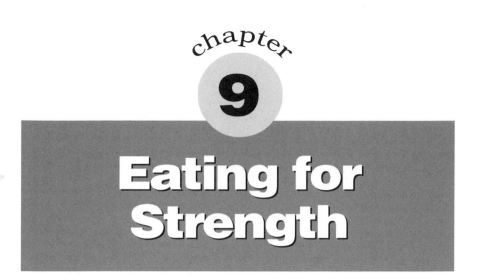

chapter

9

Eating for Strength

Your dietary habits have a major impact on your body weight, body composition, and physical health. Unfortunately, most Americans consume too many calories for the amount of activity they do. As a result, about three out of every four adults are overweight, which predisposes them to various diseases and degenerative problems. You are probably aware that excessive body fat increases the risk of heart disease, joint problems, diabetes, and many types of cancer. Yet, eating too little protein or calcium can lead to a weak musculoskeletal system, even osteoporosis. Insufficient iron in your diet may cause you to become anemic, whereas excessive sodium intake may contribute to hypertension.

Of course, eating foods high in fiber, low in fat, and rich in vitamins and minerals is essential for optimum health, as well as for disease prevention. For example, potassium, which is found in bananas and cantaloupe, is involved in every muscle contraction. Vitamins A and C, found in many fruits and vegetables, are considered important antioxidants (nutritional bodyguards) that protect us from potentially harmful chemical reactions in our body cells.

While you can consume vitamins and minerals through nutritional supplements, we strongly recommend that you do not substitute such supplements for a well-balanced diet that includes a variety of vegetables, fruits, and whole grains, as well as lean meats and low-fat dairy products. Human nutrient requirements are too complex (and too poorly understood) to be adequately supported by pills, and only a varied and well-rounded diet can provide the proper foundation for optimum nutrition. We firmly support the food categories and daily servings recommended by the United States Department of Agriculture in the Food Guide Pyramid. And remember, a well-balanced diet is not the same as a low-calorie diet designed for losing weight. Reduced calorie diets should be approved by your physician or a registered dietitian.

The Basic Nutrients

As shown in figure 9.1, the Food Guide Pyramid is high in carbohydrates, moderate in proteins, and low in fats. The carbohydrate choices are divided into grains, vegetables, and fruits. The suggested protein sources are low-fat milk products and lean meats, and the recommended fat-rich foods are vegetable oils (used sparingly). Let's consider each of the food categories more carefully.

Grains

Grains include all kinds of foods made from wheat, oats, corn, rice, and the like. Examples of grain foods are cereals, breads, pasta, pancakes, rice cakes, tortillas, bagels, muffins, cornbread, rice pudding, and chocolate cake. Obviously, some grain-based foods such as cakes, cookies, and pastries contain a lot of fat, so you should eat them sparingly.

All grains are high in carbohydrates, and some grains or parts of grains, such as wheat germ, are also good sources of protein. Whole grains are typically rich in B vitamins and fiber. Grains are plentiful and inexpensive and should be a part of every meal. In fact, the Food Guide Pyramid recommends 6 to 11 servings of grains every day. A serving is equivalent to a slice of bread or a half cup of cooked pasta, so achieving the 6 to 11 servings is not really difficult.

Refer to page 182 for sample exchange units for popular food choices within the grains category.

Food Guide Pyramid

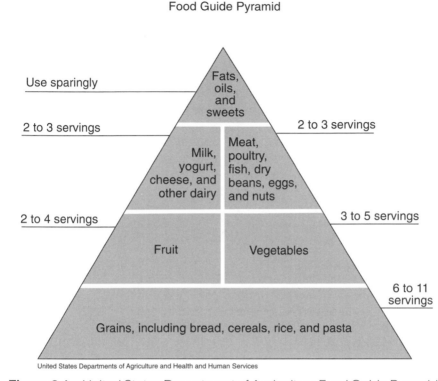

Use sparingly

2 to 3 servings

2 to 4 servings

Fats, oils, and sweets

Milk, yogurt, cheese, and other dairy

Meat, poultry, fish, dry beans, eggs, and nuts

Fruit

Vegetables

2 to 3 servings

3 to 5 servings

6 to 11 servings

Grains, including bread, cereals, rice, and pasta

United States Departments of Agriculture and Health and Human Services

Figure 9.1   United States Department of Agriculture Food Guide Pyramid.

Vegetables

Like grains, vegetables are excellent sources of carbohydrates, vitamins, and fiber. Vegetables come in all sizes, shapes, colors, and nutritional characteristics, and they are relatively low in calories. Orange vegetables are typically good sources of vitamin A and beta-carotene. This category includes carrots, sweet potatoes, and winter squash.

Green vegetables are characteristically high in vitamins B2 and folic acid. Some of the many green vegetables are peas, beans, broccoli, asparagus, spinach, and lettuce.

Red vegetables generally provide ample amounts of vitamin C. The best known vegetables in this category are tomatoes and red peppers.

Other vegetables are essentially white, at least under the skin. These include cauliflower, summer squash, potatoes, and radishes, many of which are good sources of vitamin C.

SAMPLE EXCHANGE UNITS EQUIVALENT TO ONE GRAIN SERVING

Cereals

> 1/4 c. nugget cereals (Grape Nuts)
> 1/3 c. concentrated bran cereals
> 1/2 c. cooked hot cereal (oatmeal or Cream of Wheat)
> 3/4 c. flaked cereals
> 1 1/2 c. puffed cereals

Breads

> 1/2 bagel or English muffin
> 1 slice bread
> 1 piece pita bread
> 1 tortilla

Grains

> 1/4 c. wheat germ
> 1/3 c. brown or white rice
> 1/2 c. pasta, macaroni, or noodles
> 1/2 c. hominy, barley, or grits

Snacks

> 3/4 oz. pretzels
> 3/4 oz. rice cakes
> 4 crackers (1 oz.)
> 3 c. air-popped popcorn

The Food Guide Pyramid recommends three to five daily servings of vegetables. One serving is one-half cup of any raw vegetable, except for lettuce and sprouts which require one cup per serving. Because heating reduces water content, cooked vegetables require less space than uncooked vegetables and serving sizes may be smaller. Likewise, vegetable juices are more concentrated and require only one-half cup per serving.

It is a good idea to eat some of your vegetables raw and to steam or microwave other vegetables for nutrient retention. In addition, fresh and frozen vegetables have more nutritional value and are lower in sodium than canned vegetables.

Fruit

Fruit is the counterpart to vegetables, relatively low in calories, with as much variety and nutritional value. Essentially all fruit choices are high in carbohydrates and vitamins, and many provide excellent sources of fiber.

As you probably know, citrus fruit, such as oranges, grapefruit, and lemons are loaded with vitamin C. Like orange-colored vegetables, orange-colored fruit, including cantaloupe, apricots, and papaya, are rich in vitamin A and beta-carotene.

Both green fruit, such as honeydew melon and kiwi, and red fruit, such as strawberries and cherries, are high in vitamin C.

Yellow fruit includes peaches, mangos, and pineapples, all of which are good sources of vitamin C. Fruit that is white, at least on the inside, includes apples, pears, and bananas, all of which are high in potassium.

Dried fruits are particularly nutrient dense, and the natural sweetness make them healthy substitutes for high-fat snacks such as candy bars. Raisins, dates, figs, and prunes are all superb energy sources, and prunes are the single best source of dietary fiber.

The Food Guide Pyramid recommends two to four servings of fruit every day. The chart below presents sample exchange quantities for a variety of fruits. You will notice that one serving varies considerably, depending on the type of fruit you eat. For example, it takes one-quarter of a melon or one-half of a grapefruit to equal three dates or two tablespoons of raisins. The difference is water content. Fresh fruit contains lots of water, whereas dried fruit is essentially a high-density carbohydrate. If you prefer your fruit in liquid form, one-half cup of fruit juice equals one serving, but has less fiber than whole fruit.

SAMPLE EXCHANGE UNITS EQUIVALENT TO ONE FRUIT SERVING

2 T. raisins	1 pear	1/4 melon
3 dates	3 apricots	1/2 mango
3 prunes	1/2 grapefruit	5 kumquats
1/2 c. grapes	3/4 c. pineapple	1 c. honeydew
3/4 c. berries	2 kiwi	1 1/4 c. strawberries
1 apple	1/2 pomegranate	1 1/4 c. watermelon
1 banana	1/4 canteloupe	
1 peach	1/4 papaya	

Milk Products

The Food Guide Pyramid recommends two to three daily servings of low-fat dairy products, including milk, yogurt, and cheese. These foods are excellent sources of protein and calcium. Because whole milk products are high in fat, you should be selective at the dairy counter. For example, one percent milk, low-fat yogurt, and nonfat cottage cheese offer heart healthy alternatives to higher-fat dairy selections.

Refer to the chart below for exchange units equivalent to one dairy serving. Notice that one-quarter cup of low-fat cottage cheese has similar nutritional value to one cup of one percent milk. Although there are many sources of dietary protein, you may have difficulty obtaining sufficient calcium unless you regularly consume milk products. If you have problems digesting milk (lactose intolerance), try to regularly consume other foods that are high in calcium such as tofu, leafy greens, beans, broccoli, and sesame seeds.

Meats

According to the Food Guide Pyramid, this category includes meat, poultry, fish, eggs, nuts, and dry beans. All these foods are good sources of protein, although some also contain significant amounts of fat. Table 9.1 presents sample foods in the meat category according to their fat content. You will note that how the meat is prepared has a lot to do with how much fat it provides. We'll look at this aspect in more detail in the food preparation section.

While there are differences in fat content, protein exchange units are quite consistent among the foods in the meat category. As you can see from the list on page 185, three

SAMPLE EXCHANGE UNITS EQUIVALENT TO ONE DAIRY SERVING	
1 oz. low-fat cheese	1/2 c. evaporated skim milk
1/4 c. low-fat or nonfat cottage cheese	1 c. nonfat or 1% milk
1/4 c. part-skim ricotta cheese	1 c. low-fat or nonfat yogurt
1/4 c. parmesan cheese	1 c. low-fat buttermilk

Table 9.1

MEAT GROUP FOODS
CATEGORIZED BY FAT CONTENT

Low fat	Medium fat	High fat
All fish	Chicken with skin	Beef ribs
Egg whites	Turkey with skin	Pork ribs
Chicken without skin	Roast beef	Corned beef
Turkey without skin	Roast pork	Sausage
Venison	Roast lamb	Lunch meat
Rabbit	Veal cutlet	Ground pork
Top round	Ground beef	Hot dogs
Eye of round	Steaks	Fried chicken
Sirloin tenderloin	Canned salmon	Fried fish
Flank steak	Oil-packed tuna	Nuts
Veal	Whole eggs	Peanuts
Dry beans	Pork chops	Peanut butter

SAMPLE EXCHANGE UNITS EQUIVALENT
TO ONE MEAT SERVING

3 oz. fish	1 T. peanut butter
3 oz. poultry	1/4 c. cooked dry beans
3 oz. meat (beef, poultry, lamb, etc.)	1/4 c. tuna
1 egg or 2 egg whites	1/4 c. tofu

ounces of meat, poultry, and fish (about the size of a deck of cards) have equal exchange value, as do one-quarter cup of dry beans and one-quarter cup of tuna. Try to consume two to three servings, for a total of six to nine ounces, from the meat group on a daily basis.

Fats

The smallest section of the Food Guide Pyramid is the fat group, which you should consume sparingly. Although all fats contain more than nine calories per gram, some fats are more desirable than others from a health perspective. For example, the consumption of saturated fats (such as those found in mayonnaise, butter, and sour cream) puts you at higher risk for developing heart disease than monounsaturated fats (such as those found in olive oil and canola oil) and polyunsaturated fats (such as those found in margarine and corn oil). See the chart below to determine serving equivalents for foods in the fat group.

Water: The Most Important Nutrient

Water is not included in the Food Guide Pyramid, because it contains no calories and is not technically a food. Nonetheless, it is far and away the most important nutrient for your body. Your body is mostly water (even your muscles are 80 percent water) and you can live only a few days without taking in water.

The standard recommendation is to drink eight eight-ounce glasses of water daily, and even more water is desirable when you exercise. Unfortunately, our natural thirst mechanism declines with age, so active adults should monitor their water consumption to make sure they drink at least eight glasses every day.

Because coffee, tea, diet drinks, and alcoholic beverages act as diuretics, which have a dehydrating effect, you should not count them in the daily water supply. But you may substitute other beverages for water, such as seltzer and fruit juices. Apple juice is an excellent source of potassium, and, of course, orange juice is high in vitamin C. Cranberry juice is close to

SAMPLE EXCHANGE UNITS EQUIVALENT TO ONE FAT SERVING	
1 t. butter	1 T. cream cheese
1 t. margarine	2 T. light cream cheese
1 T. diet margarine	2 T. sour cream
1 t. mayonnaise	4 T. light sour cream
1 T. diet mayonnaise	2 T. coffee creamer (liquid)
1 t. oil	
1 T. salad dressing	
2 T. diet salad dressing	

orange juice in vitamin C content and may help prevent bladder infections. Carrot juice is high in vitamin A, vitamin C, potassium, and fiber.

Three Steps to Better Nutrition

An eating program that provides all your essential nutrients but limits fat consumption requires careful food selection, substitution, and preparation. The following suggestions should help you actually implement your best intentions.

Food Selection

If you use the Food Guide Pyramid guidelines, emphasizing grains, vegetables, and fruit, along with moderate amounts of milk and meat products, your diet will be generally high in nutrition and low in fat. You should, however, select more carefully in the fat category. Because saturated fats such as those found in butter, cream, egg yolks, palm oil, and coconut oil raise blood cholesterol levels, you should consume these foods sparingly. Instead, select monounsaturated fats, such as olive and peanut oils, or polyunsaturated fats, such as safflower, sunflower, and corn oils. Mono- and polyunsaturated oils tend to lower blood cholesterol levels and may therefore help reduce the risk of heart disease.

The foods listed here and those shown in figure 9.2 contain less saturated fat than other choices in their category, so select them whenever possible:

- Fish
- Poultry without skin
- Low-fat milk, yogurt, cottage cheese
- Olive, peanut, sunflower, safflower, corn, canola oils

Note: Avoid prepared foods that contain saturated fats such as palm and coconut oils as well as hydrogenated products. The container label will indicate if a food is high in saturated fat.

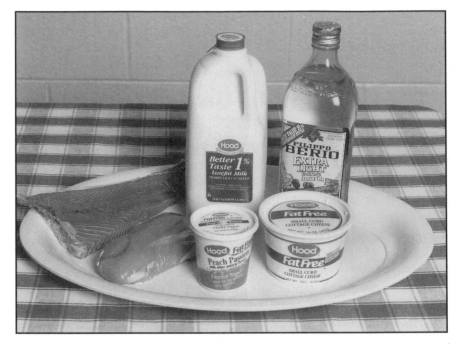

Figure 9.2 It is best to use low fat fats and to substitute monounsaturated oils when possible.

Food Substitution

You undoubtedly have certain favorite foods that you do not want to give up even though they are rich in fat. You may be surprised to discover that simple substitutions can reduce the fat content without detracting from the taste. For example, using evaporated skim milk in place of cream cuts the fat and cholesterol content by more than 65 percent. Another practical substitution is to use plain nonfat yogurt or nonfat sour cream in place of sour cream on baked potatoes. This reduces the cholesterol content by 90 percent and supplies your body with twice as much beneficial calcium.

Other useful substitutes are two egg whites in place of a whole egg, herbs rather than table salt, low-fat frozen yogurt instead of ice cream, cocoa powder in place of chocolate squares in baked goods, and lemon juice or vinegar instead of high-fat salad dressings.

If you have a sweet tooth, try eating dried fruit (raisins, dates, figs, prunes, dried apricots) in place of candy, cookies, and fat-rich baked goods. If you prefer crunchy snacks like potato chips, you may appreciate lower-fat alternatives such as pretzels (watch sodium, though), baked chips, or carrot sticks.

Food Preparation

How you prepare your food may increase or decrease the fat content. For example, frying can double and triple the calories in some foods. By using a nonfat vegetable spray or a nonstick skillet you can eliminate the fats and oils typically necessary for frying. It is also better to cook vegetables separate from meat, so that they won't absorb fats from the meat. Baked or broiled meats are recommended, and steamed or microwaved vegetables are suggested for nutrient retention. Avoid adding butter and salt to vegetables during the cooking process. If you prefer, apply these sparingly to suit individual taste once the servings are on your plate. This is because it takes less salt and fat to make food taste good after cooking than during cooking.

Summary

Healthy eating is not the same as dieting. Dieting implies a significant reduction in calories for the purpose of losing weight, usually in a short period of time. Most weight-loss diets involve unnatural eating patterns and too few nutrients for optimum physical function. Because such diets deprive you of important elements, most people cannot maintain diets very long, and they typically regain the weight they have lost soon after they discontinue the diet.

The eating pattern recommended in the United States Department of Agriculture Food Guide Pyramid is heart healthy and nutritious and can easily become part of a lifestyle that leads to improved physical well-being. You should find that a sound eating program provides plenty of energy for your strength-training workouts and essential nutrients to enhance your muscular development.

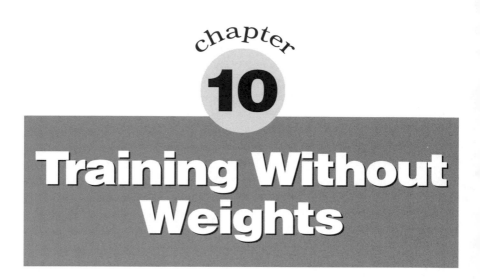

Training Without Weights

You should now understand the principles of sensible strength training and be familiar with standard machine and free-weight exercises. But maybe you don't have access to a machine training facility, or you don't feel comfortable using free weights on your own. In this chapter, we'll present simple alternatives to standard strength training with machines and free weights. But please remember that even though the exercise resistance is different, the exercise principles are essentially the same.

Strength-Training Alternatives

While we believe that machine and free-weight training offer certain advantages, you can certainly obtain good results with other forms of resistance. In fact, you can even use your own body weight as resistance. One drawback of body-weight exercises, however, is the difficulty of adjusting the resistance to your strength level. For example, on the one hand, if you are not strong enough to do a single push-up, this exercise is not appropriate. On the other hand, if at present you can perform 30 push-ups, this exercise may not be very effective for further enhancing your muscle strength. We will show you how to adapt some body-weight exercises to make them more practical and productive.

Body-weight Exercises

Each of the following exercises can be done with your body weight. We will present them in a progressive sequence from less demanding to more demanding. Be sure to breathe continuously during your body-weight exercises, exhaling during the harder upward movement phases and inhaling during the easier downward movement phases.

For Lower Strength Levels

Begin your body-weight exercise program with table push-ups, trunk curls, and quarter–knee bends. When you can complete 12 controlled repetitions in two successive workouts, progress to the next level of difficulty.

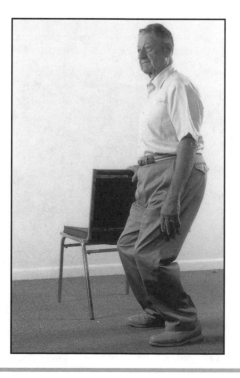

Push-Ups

Push-ups work your upper body's pushing muscles, namely, the chest, back of the arms, and shoulders. Be sure to keep your back straight in all the push-up exercises.

Table Push-Ups: Stand about four feet from a table, and place your hands slightly more than shoulder-width apart on the table edge. Lower your torso slowly until your chest is near the table, pause momentarily, and push up to the starting position (see figure 10.1). For safety, make sure the table is stable or braced against a wall.

Floor Push-Ups: To do traditional floor push-ups, place your hands slightly more than shoulder-width apart on the floor, maintaining a straight body posture. Lower your torso slowly until your chest is near the floor, pause momentarily, and push up to the starting position (see figure 10.2). If the straight

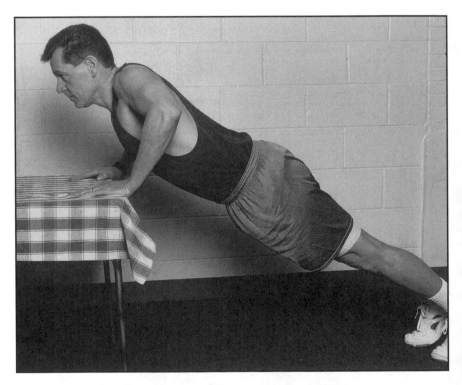

Figure 10.1 Table push-ups are one way to use your body weight in training.

body position makes it too difficult for you to complete at least eight repetitions, do the push-ups from your knees to reduce the resistance.

You may also vary your hand position to change the training emphasis. Placing your hands farther apart places more stress on the chest muscles, and placing your hands closer together places more emphasis on the back-of-arm muscles.

Chair Push-Ups: When you can complete 12 to 16 controlled push-ups, you may make this exercise more difficult by putting your feet on a stable chair or box. Place your hands slightly wider than your shoulders on the floor, maintaining a straight body posture. Lower your torso slowly until your chest is near the floor, pause momentarily, and push up to the starting position (see figure 10.3).

Trunk Curls

Properly performed trunk curls address the abdominal muscles in the front (rectus abdominis) and sides (external and internal obliques) of your midsection. Be sure you feel comfortable with the trunk curl before you advance to the more challenging abdominal exercises. As you add more repetitions, making the trunk curl sets more difficult, a greater amount of work is required.

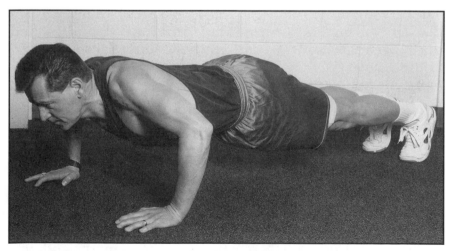

Figure 10.2 The floor push-up is an excellent upper body exercise.

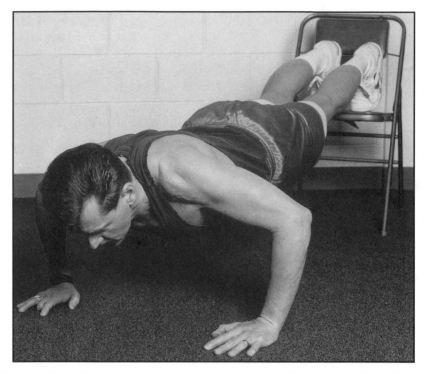

Figure 10.3 When you are ready, you may want to increase the difficulty of your workout by trying chair push-ups.

Trunk Curl With Bent Knees: Lie face up with your knees bent and your feet flat on the floor. Place your hands loosely on the sides of your head to help keep your head and neck in a neutral position during each repetition. Curl your shoulders and upper back slowly off the floor, until your lower back is pressed firmly against the floor. Pause momentarily and return slowly to the starting position (see figure 10.4).

Trunk Curl With Knee Pull: This exercise is very similar to the basic trunk curl with one additional component. As you curl your shoulders and upper back up, pull your left knee back and try to touch it with your left elbow. Pause momentarily, and then return to the starting position. On your next repetition, pull your right knee back and try to touch it with your right elbow. Continue to alternate leg lifts on each trunk curl (see figure 10.5). This exercise provides resistance from both the upper and lower body, placing more stress on the abdominal and hip flexor muscles.

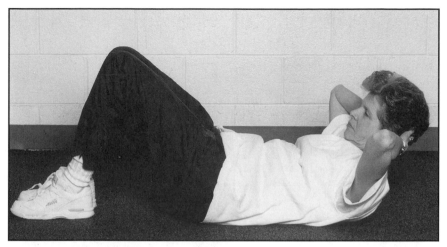

Figure 10.4 To work your abdominal muscles, try bent-knee trunk curls.

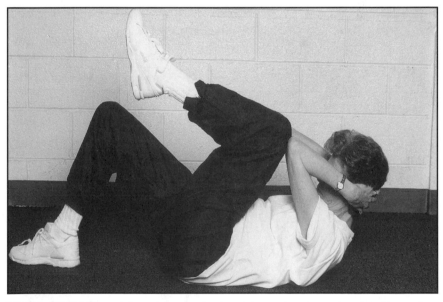

Figure 10.5 To add resistance to bent-knee trunk curls, do alternating knee pulls.

Twisting Trunk Curl With Legs on Chair: Assume your basic trunk curl starting position, but place your legs on a stable chair or box. Curl your shoulders and upper back slowly off the floor until your lower back is pressed firmly against the floor and alternately twist to the left or right. Pause momentarily, then return slowly to the starting position. Repeat the twist, but to the opposite side. The alternating twists emphasize the muscles on each side of your midsection as well as the front abdominals (see figure 10.6).

Knee Bends

Knee bends engage both your front- and back-of-thigh muscles. You should be somewhat familiar with this exercise if you performed the leg squat test in chapter 2. The difference is that this exercise is done without a chair, although you may hold onto a chair for balance if necessary. Another option is to keep your back in contact with a smooth wall as you move down and up. Because this is a relatively simple exercise, the variations involve progressively greater movement range and progressively slower movement speed. If you have no orthopedic problems with your knees or hips, knee bends are safe for you to perform. However, if you experience any pain or instability, you should not perform these exercises.

Quarter–Knee Bends: With your feet slightly more than shoulder-width apart and your torso erect, lower your hips downward and backward to a one-quarter–knee bend position. Pause momentarily and return to the starting position.

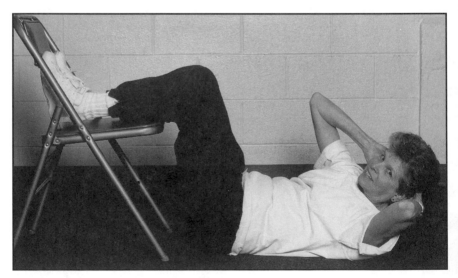

Figure 10.6 The twisting trunk curl with legs on a chair emphasizes more of your midsection muscles.

Take four full seconds (two seconds down, two seconds up) for each repetition. Try to keep your feet flat on the floor throughout the exercise (see figure 10.7).

Half–Knee Bends: This exercise is performed in the same manner as quarter–knee bends except that you lower your hips downward and backward to a one-half–knee bend position. Take six full seconds (four seconds down, two seconds up) for each repetition (see figure 10.8).

Three-Quarter–Knee Bends: This exercise is simply a more demanding version of the half–knee bend. Lower your hips downward and backward to a three-quarter–knee bend position, taking four seconds on the down movement and four seconds on the up movement (eight seconds each repetition).

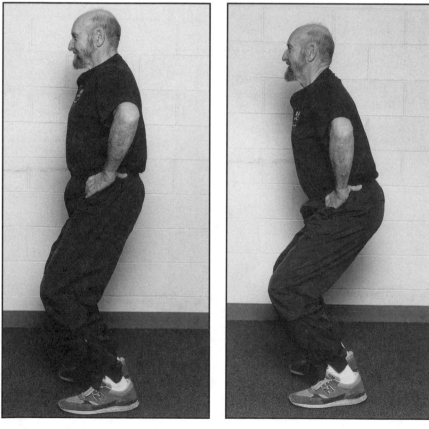

Figure 10.7 Quarter knee-bend.   **Figure 10.8** Half-knee bend.

Figure 10.9 illustrates the down position of the three-quarter–knee bend exercise.

Pull-Ups

Pull-ups are effective for developing the upper back and front-of-arm muscles, but many people find this exercise too difficult. However, because our muscles are stronger in lowering movements than lifting movements, almost everyone should be able to do these pull-up variations. In all pull-up exercises, use an underhand grip and keep your back straight and your head up.

Step Box Pull-Up—Lowering Only: Grasp the bar with palms toward you, about shoulder-width apart. Step onto the box so that your chin is above the bar, and lower your body slowly until your elbows are extended. Step onto the box again to resume the starting position (see figure 10.10).

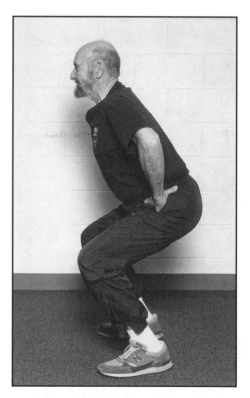

Figure 10.9   Three-quarter knee-bends add intensity to your workout.

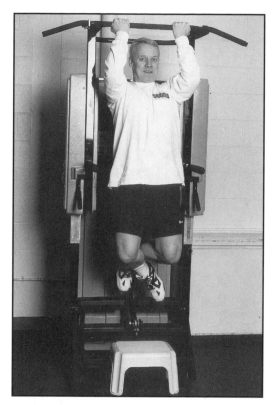

Figure 10.10 Step box pull-ups can be done by people of varying strength levels.

Step Box Pull-Up—Leg Assist: Grasp the bar with palms facing you, about shoulder-width apart. Step onto the box, then bend your knees so that your elbows are nearly extended. Use your legs to help lift your body in the upward phase of the pull-up (see figure 10.11). Lower your body without leg assistance.

Partial Pull-Up: Assume your standard grip with palms facing you and use the box to help you acquire a position with your chin above the bar. Lower your body slowly until your elbows are one-quarter extended, then pull up to the starting position (see figure 10.12). As you become stronger you may lower your body until your elbows are extended half of the way. The next step is a three-quarter repetition, and the final stage involves complete elbow extension for a full-range pull-up.

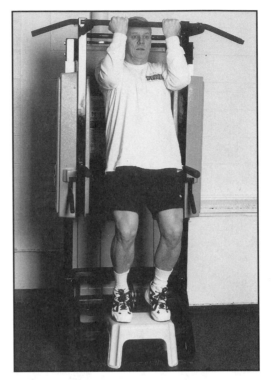

Figure 10.11 Using your legs for pull-up assistance can enhance the strengthening process.

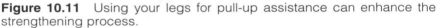

Homemade Resistance Equipment

If you prefer not to do body-weight exercises, you may easily devise homemade resistance equipment similar to free weights. For example, a quart container filled with water can function as a two-pound dumbbell, a half-gallon container of water can serve as a four-pound dumbbell, and a gallon container of water provides eight pounds of weight. But be sure to secure the cap or you may lose some of your resistance as you exercise! Although not quite as convenient or easy to handle, you may use homemade resistance equipment to do any of the dumbbell exercises presented in chapter 5.

Resistance Bands

Another alternative to traditional strength-training equipment is resistance bands. They are made from elastic material,

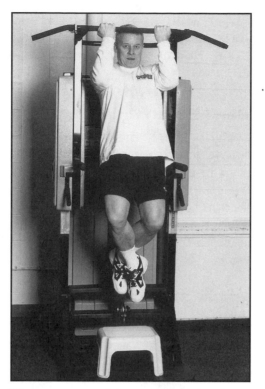

Figure 10.12 When you are ready, try a partial pull-up.

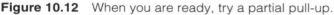

providing resistance as you stretch them. The bands come in different thicknesses and offer varying levels of resistance. You should, therefore, have several resistance bands to accommodate smaller and larger muscle groups and to progressively increase training intensity in a systematic manner.

The advantages of resistance bands include their convenience, low cost, and versatility. They are also useful when traveling, as they can easily be packed in a garment bag or briefcase. You can perform essentially any movement pattern and mimic most of the free-weight exercises. We recommend doing your band exercises with slow movement speed and full movement range. When you can complete 12 repetitions of an exercise, try using the next higher resistance level.

Resistance Band Squats

This exercise involves both the front- and back-of-thigh muscles. Stand with both feet squarely on the resistance band, slightly more than shoulder-width apart. Grasp the ends of the bands with your hands so that the band is taut in the three-quarter–knee bend position. Extend your knees and hips until you are nearly standing, then return slowly to the starting position (see figure 10.13).

Resistance Band Bench Press

Like the free-weight bench press, this exercise uses your chest, back-of-arm, and front shoulder muscles. We recommend that you sit in a sturdy chair and place the resistance band behind the chair back. Hold the ends of the band with your hands near your chest so that it is taut. Push your hands forward until your arms are almost straight in front of you, then return slowly to the starting position (see figure 10.14).

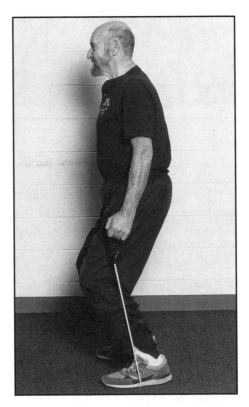

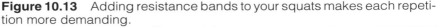

Figure 10.13   Adding resistance bands to your squats makes each repetition more demanding.

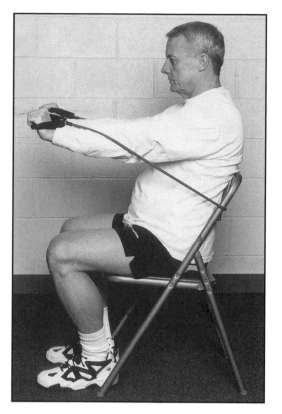

Figure 10.14 A variation of the bench press can be performed using resistance bands.

Resistance Band Seated Rows

This exercise works your upper back, front-of-arm, and rear shoulder muscles from a stable, floor-supported position. Sit on the floor with your legs straight and your torso erect. Place the elastic band around your shoes and grasp the ends with your arms extended straight in front of you so that the band is taut. While maintaining an erect torso, pull your hands to your chest, pause momentarily, and return the handles slowly to the starting position (see figure 10.15).

These three resistance band exercises address most of your major muscle groups, providing a good basic workout. One caution, however: Make sure the band is carefully secured before stretching it.

"I had polio as a child. In 1994, having bad pain in both hips and trouble walking . . . I went to a physical [therapist] . . .He gave up after three months.

Then [hip and back X rays] showed serious osteoarthritis in both hips . . . and descending spondylitis of the spine. . . . I started going to Dr. Wayne Westcott's strength-training class at the Quincy, Massachusetts YMCA, where I eventually booked private lessons with Skip Tull, who specializes with people having severe limitations. After eight months . . . weight training two or three times a week, it's a miracle—not much pain. First time in five years! My walking gait is noticeably better. . . . I also don't feel as sluggish."

—Evelyn B. Spaulding, age 71

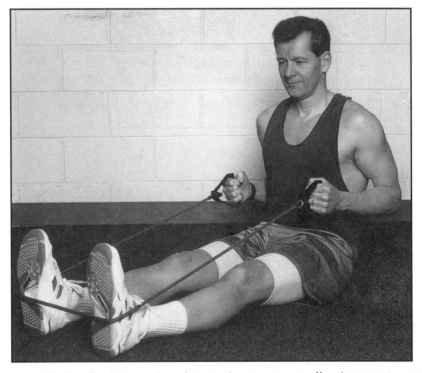

Figure 10.15 Resistance band seated rows are an effective way to work your upper back, front-of-arm and rear shoulder muscles.

Strength-Training Adjuncts

In addition to developing more muscular strength, you may want to improve your cardiovascular endurance and joint flexibility.

Endurance Exercise

You can increase your cardiovascular endurance by doing one or more aerobic activities, such as walking, cycling, or swimming. If you prefer to exercise indoors, you may want to start with stationary cycling or treadmill walking. As shown in figure 10.16, the cycle supports your body weight and allows you to pedal against as much or as little resistance as you desire.

Treadmill walking provides similar cardiovascular benefit, but requires you to keep pace with a moving track. This may take a little practice at first but should soon become second nature. Although your body weight provides the resistance, you may adjust the track speed and the treadmill elevation to match your fitness level (see figure 10.17).

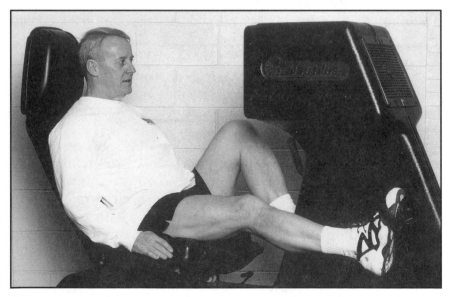

Figure 10.16   If you prefer indoor aerobic activities, weight supported cycle exercise may be ideal.

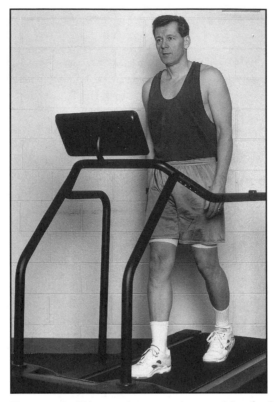

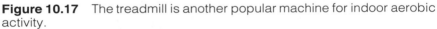

Figure 10.17 The treadmill is another popular machine for indoor aerobic activity.

Gradually work your way up to 20 minutes or more of continuous endurance exercises, at least three days each week. You should train at a moderate effort level, which means you can still talk while you exercise.

Your endurance exercises session should begin easily for a smooth transition from rest to activity. So warm up for at least five minutes. Likewise, you should end your endurance session with five or more minutes of easy cycling or walking. Remember, the cool-down period provides a safe and gradual return to resting blood circulation. If you are training properly, you should finish your endurance exercises feeling invigorated rather than exhausted.

As we noted in chapter 6, if you do your strength training and endurance exercises in the same workout, the activity order is up to you. Research has shown similar strength gains whether you do your endurance exercises before or after your strength training.

Flexibility Exercise

You can enhance your joint flexibility by doing static stretching exercises. To perform a static stretch, move slowly into the desired position and hold the stretch for about 15 to 30 seconds. Perhaps the best overall stretch is the figure-4 stretch, so named because your body position resembles a "4" (see figure 10.18).

Begin this stretch by sitting on the floor with your right leg straight and your left leg bent so that your left foot touches your right thigh. Next, reach your right hand forward and grasp your foot, ankle, or lower leg until you feel a gentle stretch. (Never stretch until it hurts!) Now hold the stretched position for 15 to 30 seconds. Do not bounce. Reverse your leg position, reach your left hand toward your left foot, ankle, or

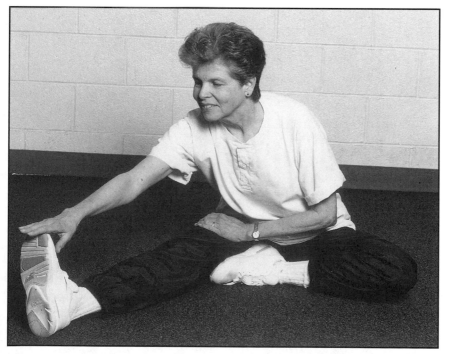

Figure 10.18 The figure-4 stretch enhances joint flexibility.

lower leg and hold the stretched position for 15 to 30 seconds. You should feel this stretch in the back of your lower leg, the back of your thigh, your lower back, and your shoulder. We recommend that you do the figure-4 stretch after you are warmed up, because your muscles stretch more easily when they are warm. Several minutes of walking or cycling serve this purpose well.

Summary

A combined program of strength training, endurance, activity and stretching exercises is hard to beat for improving your overall physical fitness. Within a few weeks you should look, feel, and function better. As we state in chapter 1, we know of no better way to develop and maintain a robust body and an active lifestyle throughout the midlife years.

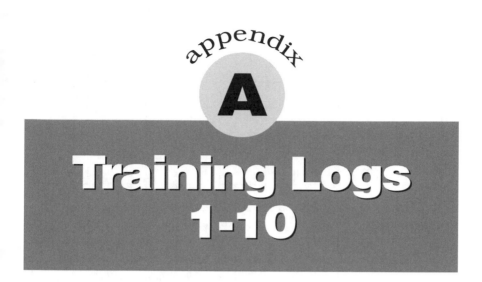

appendix

A

Training Logs
1-10

Training Log 1
Machine Exercises—Weeks 1 and 2

Name _____

Order	Exercise	Reps./Sets	Set	Week # ___ Day 1			Day 2			Day 3			Week # ___ Day 1			Day 2			Day 3		
				1	2	3	1	2	3	1	2	3	1	2	3	1	2	3	1	2	3
1	Leg press		Wt.																		
			Reps.																		
2	Chest press		Wt.																		
			Reps.																		
3	Compound row		Wt.																		
			Reps.																		
4	Abdominal curl		Wt.																		
			Reps.																		
5	Back extension		Wt.																		
			Reps.																		
6			Wt.																		
			Reps.																		
7			Wt.																		
			Reps.																		
8			Wt.																		
			Reps.																		
9			Wt.																		
			Reps.																		
10			Wt.																		
			Reps.																		
11			Wt.																		
			Reps.																		
12			Wt.																		
			Reps.																		
Body weight																					
Date																					
Comments																					

Training Log 2
Free-Weight Exercises—Weeks 1 and 2

Name _____

Order	Exercise	Reps./Sets	Set	Week # ___ Day 1			Day 2			Day 3			Week # ___ Day 1			Day 2			Day 3		
				1	2	3	1	2	3	1	2	3	1	2	3	1	2	3	1	2	3
1	Dumbbell squat		Wt.																		
			Reps.																		
2	Dumbbell bench press		Wt.																		
			Reps.																		
3	Dumbbell one-arm row		Wt.																		
			Reps.																		
4	Dumbbell seated press		Wt.																		
			Reps.																		
5	Trunk curl		Wt.																		
			Reps.																		
6			Wt.																		
			Reps.																		
7			Wt.																		
			Reps.																		
8			Wt.																		
			Reps.																		
9			Wt.																		
			Reps.																		
10			Wt.																		
			Reps.																		
11			Wt.																		
			Reps.																		
12			Wt.																		
			Reps.																		
Body weight																					
Date																					
Comments																					

Training Log 3
Machine Exercises—Weeks 3 and 4

Name _____

Order	Exercise	Reps./Sets	Set	Week # ___ Day 1			Day 2			Day 3			Week # ___ Day 1			Day 2			Day 3		
				1	2	3	1	2	3	1	2	3	1	2	3	1	2	3	1	2	3
1	Leg press		Wt.																		
			Reps.																		
2	Hip adduction		Wt.																		
			Reps.																		
3	Hip abduction		Wt.																		
			Reps.																		
4	Chest press		Wt.																		
			Reps.																		
5	Compound row		Wt.																		
			Reps.																		
6	Abdominal curl		Wt.																		
			Reps.																		
7	Back extension		Wt.																		
			Reps.																		
8			Wt.																		
			Reps.																		
9			Wt.																		
			Reps.																		
10			Wt.																		
			Reps.																		
11			Wt.																		
			Reps.																		
12			Wt.																		
			Reps.																		
Body weight																					
Date																					
Comments																					

Training Log 4
Free-Weight Exercises—Weeks 3 and 4

Name _____

Order	Exercise	Reps. Sets	Set	Week # ___ Day 1			Day 2			Day 3			Week # ___ Day 1			Day 2			Day 3		
				1	2	3	1	2	3	1	2	3	1	2	3	1	2	3	1	2	3
1	Dumbbell squat		Wt.																		
			Reps.																		
2	Dumbbell bench press		Wt.																		
			Reps.																		
3	Dumbbell one-arm row		Wt.																		
			Reps.																		
4	Dumbbell seated press		Wt.																		
			Reps.																		
5	Dumbbell curl		Wt.																		
			Reps.																		
6	Dumbbell overhead triceps extension		Wt.																		
			Reps.																		
7	Trunk curl		Wt.																		
			Reps.																		
8			Wt.																		
			Reps.																		
9			Wt.																		
			Reps.																		
10			Wt.																		
			Reps.																		
11			Wt.																		
			Reps.																		
12			Wt.																		
			Reps.																		
Body weight																					
Date																					
Comments																					

Training Log 5
Machine Exercises—Weeks 5 and 6

Name

Order	Exercise	Reps. Sets	Set	Week # Day 1 1 2 3	Day 2 1 2 3	Day 3 1 2 3	Week # Day 1 1 2 3	Day 2 1 2 3	Day 3 1 2 3
1	Leg press		Wt. Reps.						
2	Hip adduction		Wt. Reps.						
3	Hip abduction		Wt. Reps.						
4	Chest press		Wt. Reps.						
5	Compound row		Wt. Reps.						
6	Triceps extension		Wt. Reps.						
7	Biceps curl		Wt. Reps.						
8	Abdominal curl		Wt. Reps.						
9	Back extension		Wt. Reps.						
10			Wt. Reps.						
11			Wt. Reps.						
12			Wt. Reps.						
Body weight									
Date									
Comments									

Training Log 6
Free-Weight Exercises—Weeks 5 and 6

Name _____

Order	Exercise	Reps./Sets	Set / Wt./Reps.	Week # Day 1 (1,2,3)			Day 2 (1,2,3)			Day 3 (1,2,3)			Week # Day 1 (1,2,3)			Day 2 (1,2,3)			Day 3 (1,2,3)		
1	Dumbbell squat		Wt.																		
			Reps.																		
2	Dumbbell bench press		Wt.																		
			Reps.																		
3	Dumbbell one-arm row		Wt.																		
			Reps.																		
4	Dumbbell seated press		Wt.																		
			Reps.																		
5	Dumbbell curl		Wt.																		
			Reps.																		
6	Dumbbell overhead triceps extension		Wt.																		
			Reps.																		
7	Trunk curl		Wt.																		
			Reps.																		
8	Dumbbell shrug		Wt.																		
			Reps.																		
9	Dumbbell heel raise		Wt.																		
			Reps.																		
10			Wt.																		
			Reps.																		
11			Wt.																		
			Reps.																		
12			Wt.																		
			Reps.																		
Body weight																					
Date																					
Comments																					

Training Log 7
Machine Exercises—Weeks 7 and 8

Name _____

Order	Exercise	Reps. / Sets	Set	Week #									Week #								
				Day 1			Day 2			Day 3			Day 1			Day 2			Day 3		
				1	2	3	1	2	3	1	2	3	1	2	3	1	2	3	1	2	3
1	Leg press		Wt.																		
			Reps.																		
2	Hip adduction		Wt.																		
			Reps.																		
3	Hip abduction		Wt.																		
			Reps.																		
4	Chest crossover		Wt.																		
			Reps.																		
5	Super-pullover		Wt.																		
			Reps.																		
6	Lateral raise		Wt.																		
			Reps.																		
7	Triceps extension		Wt.																		
			Reps.																		
8	Biceps curl		Wt.																		
			Reps.																		
9	Abdominal curl		Wt.																		
			Reps.																		
10	Back extension		Wt.																		
			Reps.																		
11			Wt.																		
			Reps.																		
12			Wt.																		
			Reps.																		
Body weight																					
Date																					
Comments																					

Training Log 8
Free-Weight Exercises—Weeks 7 and 8

Name _____

Order	Exercise	Reps.		Week # ____ Day 1			Day 2			Day 3			Week # ____ Day 1			Day 2			Day 3		
		Sets	Set	1	2	3	1	2	3	1	2	3	1	2	3	1	2	3	1	2	3
1	Dumbbell squat		Wt.																		
			Reps.																		
2	Dumbbell bench press		Wt.																		
			Reps.																		
3	Dumbbell chest fly		Wt.																		
			Reps.																		
4	Dumbbell one-arm row		Wt.																		
			Reps.																		
5	Dumbbell seated press		Wt.																		
			Reps.																		
6	Dumbbell curl		Wt.																		
			Reps.																		
7	Dumbbell overhead triceps extension		Wt.																		
			Reps.																		
8	Trunk curl		Wt.																		
			Reps.																		
9	Dumbbell shrug		Wt.																		
			Reps.																		
10	Dumbbell heel raise		Wt.																		
			Reps.																		
11			Wt.																		
			Reps.																		
12			Wt.																		
			Reps.																		
	Body weight																				
	Date																				
	Comments																				

Training Log 9
Machine Exercises—Weeks 9 and 10

Name _____

Order	Exercise	Reps./Sets	Set	Week # Day 1 1	2	3	Day 2 1	2	3	Day 3 1	2	3	Week # Day 1 1	2	3	Day 2 1	2	3	Day 3 1	2	3
1	Leg extension		Wt.																		
			Reps.																		
2	Leg curl		Wt.																		
			Reps.																		
3	Hip adduction		Wt.																		
			Reps.																		
4	Hip abduction		Wt.																		
			Reps.																		
5	Chest crossover		Wt.																		
			Reps.																		
6	Super-pullover		Wt.																		
			Reps.																		
7	Lateral raise		Wt.																		
			Reps.																		
8	Triceps extension		Wt.																		
			Reps.																		
9	Biceps curl		Wt.																		
			Reps.																		
10	Abdominal curl		Wt.																		
			Reps.																		
11	Back extension		Wt.																		
			Reps.																		
12			Wt.																		
			Reps.																		
Body weight																					
Date																					
Comments																					

Training Log 10
Free-Weight Exercises—Weeks 9 and 10

Name _____

Order	Exercise	Reps. Sets	Set	Week #___ Day 1 1 2 3	Day 2 1 2 3	Day 3 1 2 3	Week #___ Day 1 1 2 3	Day 2 1 2 3	Day 3 1 2 3
1	Dumbbell squat		Wt.						
			Reps.						
2	Dumbbell bench press		Wt.						
			Reps.						
3	Dumbbell chest fly		Wt.						
			Reps.						
4	Lat pull-down		Wt.						
			Reps.						
5	Dumbbell seated press		Wt.						
			Reps.						
6	Dumbbell curl		Wt.						
			Reps.						
7	Triceps press-down		Wt.						
			Reps.						
8	Trunk curl		Wt.						
			Reps.						
9	Dumbbell shrug		Wt.						
			Reps.						
10	Dumbbell heel raise		Wt.						
			Reps.						
11			Wt.						
			Reps.						
12			Wt.						
			Reps.						
Body weight									
Date									
Comments									

219

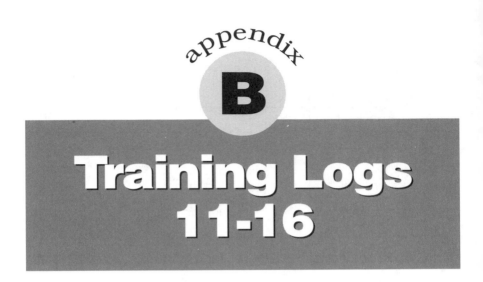

appendix

B

Training Logs 11-16

Training Log 11
Machine Exercises—Muscle Size Development

Name _____

Order	Exercise	Reps. / Sets	Set	Week # — Day 1			Day 2			Day 3			Week # — Day 1			Day 2			Day 3		
				1	2	3	1	2	3	1	2	3	1	2	3	1	2	3	1	2	3
1	Leg extension		Wt.																		
			Reps.																		
2	Leg curl		Wt.																		
			Reps.																		
3	Chest crossover		Wt.																		
			Reps.																		
4	Chest press		Wt.																		
			Reps.																		
5	Compound row		Wt.																		
			Reps.																		
6	Lateral raise		Wt.																		
			Reps.																		
7	Triceps extension		Wt.																		
			Reps.																		
8	Biceps curl		Wt.																		
			Reps.																		
9	Weight-assisted pull-ups		Wt.																		
			Reps.																		
10	Back extension		Wt.																		
			Reps.																		
11	Abdominal curl		Wt.																		
			Reps.																		
12			Wt.																		
			Reps.																		
	Body weight																				
	Date																				
	Comments																				

Training Log 12
Free-Weight Exercises—Muscle Size Development

Name _____

Order	Exercise	Reps. / Sets	Set	Week # — Day 1 (1)	Day 1 (2)	Day 1 (3)	Day 2 (1)	Day 2 (2)	Day 2 (3)	Day 3 (1)	Day 3 (2)	Day 3 (3)	Week # — Day 1 (1)	Day 1 (2)	Day 1 (3)	Day 2 (1)	Day 2 (2)	Day 2 (3)	Day 3 (1)	Day 3 (2)	Day 3 (3)
1	Squat*		Wt.																		
			Reps.																		
2	Bench press*		Wt.																		
			Reps.																		
3	Dumbbell chest fly		Wt.																		
			Reps.																		
4	Dumbbell one-arm row		Wt.																		
			Reps.																		
5	Dumbbell seated press		Wt.																		
			Reps.																		
6	Dumbbell lateral raise		Wt.																		
			Reps.																		
7	Barbell curl		Wt.																		
			Reps.																		
8	Dumbbell concentration curl		Wt.																		
			Reps.																		
9	Dumbbell overhead triceps extension		Wt.																		
			Reps.																		
10	Barbell shrug		Wt.																		
			Reps.																		
11			Wt.																		
			Reps.																		
12			Wt.																		
			Reps.																		

Body weight

Date

Comments

Name _____

Training Log 13
Machine Exercises—Strength Development

Order	Exercise	Reps. Sets	Set	Week # ___ Day 1 (1, 2, 3)	Day 2 (1, 2, 3)	Day 3 (1, 2, 3)	Week # ___ Day 1 (1, 2, 3)	Day 2 (1, 2, 3)	Day 3 (1, 2, 3)
1	Leg press		Wt. / Reps.						
2	Heel raise		Wt. / Reps.						
3	Chest press		Wt. / Reps.						
4	Compound row		Wt. / Reps.						
5	Lateral raise		Wt. / Reps.						
6	Triceps extension		Wt. / Reps.						
7	Biceps curl		Wt. / Reps.						
8	Back extension		Wt. / Reps.						
9	Abdominal curl		Wt. / Reps.						
10			Wt. / Reps.						
11			Wt. / Reps.						
12			Wt. / Reps.						
	Body weight								
	Date								
	Comments								

Training Log 14
Free-weight Exercises—Strength Development

Name

Order	Exercise	Reps. Sets	Set		Week # ___ Day 1			Day 2			Day 3			Week # ___ Day 1			Day 2			Day 3		
				1	2	3	1	2	3	1	2	3	1	2	3	1	2	3	1	2	3	
1	Squat*		Wt.																			
			Reps.																			
2	Heel raise*		Wt.																			
			Reps.																			
3	Bench press*		Wt.																			
			Reps.																			
4	Dumbbell one-arm row		Wt.																			
			Reps.																			
5	Dumbbell seated press		Wt.																			
			Reps.																			
6	Barbell curl		Wt.																			
			Reps.																			
7	Dumbbell overhead triceps extension		Wt.																			
			Reps.																			
8	Trunk curl		Wt.																			
			Reps.																			
9			Wt.																			
			Reps.																			
10			Wt.																			
			Reps.																			
11			Wt.																			
			Reps.																			
12			Wt.																			
			Reps.																			
Body weight																						
Date																						
Comments																						

Name _____

Training Log 15
Machine Exercises—Muscle Endurance

Order	Exercise	Reps. Sets	Set	Week # ___ Day 1 1	2	3	Day 2 1	2	3	Day 3 1	2	3	Week # ___ Day 1 1	2	3	Day 2 1	2	3	Day 3 1	2	3
1	Leg extension		Wt.																			
			Reps.																			
2	Leg curl		Wt.																			
			Reps.																			
3	Hip abduction		Wt.																			
			Reps.																			
4	Hip adduction		Wt.																			
			Reps.																			
5	Chest crossover		Wt.																			
			Reps.																			
6	Super-pullover		Wt.																			
			Reps.																			
7	Lateral raise		Wt.																			
			Reps.																			
8	Triceps extension		Wt.																			
			Reps.																			
9	Biceps curl		Wt.																			
			Reps.																			
10	Rotary torso		Wt.																			
			Reps.																			
11			Wt.																			
			Reps.																			
12			Wt.																			
			Reps.																			
Body weight																						
Date																						
Comments																						

Training Log 16
Free-Weight Exercises—Muscle Endurance

Name _____

Order	Exercise	Reps. Sets	Set	Week # Day 1 1	2	3	Day 2 1	2	3	Day 3 1	2	3	Week # Day 1 1	2	3	Day 2 1	2	3	Day 3 1	2	3
1	Squat*		Wt.																			
			Reps.																			
2	Heel raise*		Wt.																			
			Reps.																			
3	Bench press*		Wt.																			
			Reps.																			
4	Dumbbell chest fly		Wt.																			
			Reps.																			
5	Dumbbell one-arm row		Wt.																			
			Reps.																			
6	Dumbbell seated press		Wt.																			
			Reps.																			
7	Barbell curl		Wt.																			
			Reps.																			
8	Dumbbell overhead triceps extension		Wt.																			
			Reps.																			
9	Barbell shrug		Wt.																			
			Reps.																			
10	Trunk curl		Wt.																			
			Reps.																			
11			Wt.																			
			Reps.																			
12			Wt.																			
			Reps.																			
	Body weight																					
	Date																					
	Comments																					

226

Index

About the Authors

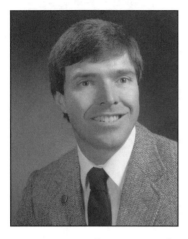

With more than 30 years in strength training as an athlete, coach, teacher, professor, researcher, writer, and speaker, Wayne Westcott, PhD, is recognized as a leading authority on fitness. He is the fitness research director at the South Shore YMCA in Massachusetts, where he developed a model strength-fitness facility and training program rated the "Best Buy in the United States" by *Fitness Magazine* in 1995.

Westcott has served as a strength training consultant for numerous organizations and programs, including Nautilus, the President's Council on Physical Fitness and Sports, the National Sports Performance Association, the International Association of Fitness Professionals (IDEA), the American Council on Exercise, the YMCA of the USA, and the National Youth Sports Safety Foundation. He was awarded the IDEA Lifetime Achievement Award in 1993 and was honored with a Healthy American Fitness Leader Award in 1995.

Westcott is the author of several books on strength training, including *Building Strength and Stamina* and *Strength Fitness: Physiological Principles and Training Techniques*, a text used by physical education and exercise science majors for more than 15 years. Westcott has also written a weekly fitness column since 1986 for one of Boston's largest newspapers. The strength training advisor and fitness columnist for *Prevention* magazine, he also has served on the editorial boards of *Prevention, Shape, Men's Health, Fitness, Club Industry, American Fitness Quarterly,* and *Nautilus.*

Westcott lives in Abington, Massachusetts, with his wife, Claudia. He enjoys strength training, running, cycling, gardening, and volunteer work.

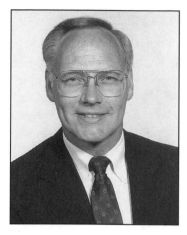

Thomas R. Baechle, EdD, CSCS, is the executive director of the NSCA Certification Commission, the certifying body for the National Strength and Conditioning Association (NSCA). He is cofounder, past president, and former director of education of the NSCA, and in 1985 was named its Strength and Conditioning Professional of the Year. Dr. Baechle also is the chair of the Department of Exercise Science at Creighton University, where he has received several honors, including an Excellence in Teaching Award.

For 16 years Dr. Baechle competed successfully in weightlifting and powerlifting, setting various Midwest records. For more than 20 years he coached collegiate powerlifting teams and taught weight training classes. Dr. Baechle also holds certifications as a Level I weightlifting coach (United States Weightlifting Federation), a Strength and Conditioning Specialist and Personal Trainer (NSCA), and an Exercise Test Technologist and Exercise Specialist (ACSM). He is a member of NSCA, ACSM, the American Alliance for Health, Physical Education, Recreation and Dance (AAHPERD), and is the current president-elect of the National Organization for Competency Assurance (NOCA). Dr. Baechle has authored several books, including the very popular *Weight Training: Steps to Success* and *Fitness Weight Training* texts, and he served as the editor of *Essentials of Strength Training and Conditioning*, regarded as the most comprehensive text in its field.

Baechle lives in Omaha, Nebraska, with his wife Susan and two sons, Todd and Clark. He enjoys woodworking and doing crafts.